I see in Dr. Max Gerson one of the most eminent geniuses in the history of medicine. Many of his basic ideas have been adopted without having his name connected with them. He has achieved more than seemed possible under adverse conditions. He leaves a legacy which commands attention and that will assure him his due place. Those whom he cured will attest to the truth of his ideas.

—*Albert Schweitzer*

GW00645176

Healing Arthritis

THE GERSON WAY

Healing Arthritis

THE GERSON WAY

BASED ON THE RESEARCH OF

Dr. Max Gerson

Charlotte Gerson

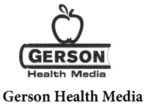

Gerson Health Media

Gerson Health Media
316 Mid Valley Center #230
Carmel, CA 93923
www.gersonmedia.com

ISBN-10: 1937 92009 7
ISBN-13: 978 1937 92009 8

The marks Gerson, Gerson Therapy and Gerson Institute are trademarks and/or service marks owned and proprietary to the Gerson Institute, San Diego, California, and are covered by appropriate domestic and/or foreign registration and/or protective laws. All other trademarks and/or service marks referred to herein are owned by and/or proprietary to their respective owners.

President of Gerson Media & Editor in Chief: Howard Straus
Publishing Supervisor & Design Coordinator: Sensei Bill Handel

Interior design, editing and production by Joanne Shwed, Backspace Ink, Pacifica, CA (www.backspaceink.com).

Cover design created by 1106 Design, Phoenix, AZ (602) 866-3226 (www.1106design.com).

To contact the Gerson Institute, please go to www.gerson.org, or call (858) 694-0707.

In Italy, contact Margaret Straus at Associazione.Gerson@gmail.com.

For other European countries, contact the Gerson Health Centre in Hungary at info@gerson.hu.

For an up-to-date list of Gerson Therapy Resources, please visit www.gerson.org.

Contents

Acknowledgements

This book is above all a tribute to my father, Dr. Max Gerson. He was not just a doctor but a true healer. He deeply understood the basic organization of the incredibly complex and wonderful organism that is the human body, and through his genius he learned how to restore and heal those who were failing. He was not only a healer, but he hoped to bring healing to all the world, to end disease and suffering.

Building on his vast knowledge and experience, we have often been able to bring complete healing, a return of life and health, to those who were once pronounced "incurable" and who faced long years of suffering or death. In this volume, we aim to bring the details of his approach to those who will use it to return to happy and productive lives.

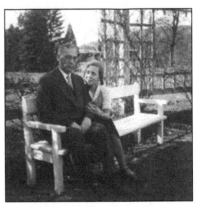

Max and Charlotte Gerson

In the past 50 years, the world has changed, conditions have worsened and the healing knowledge has had to be adapted to these changes. It has taken many people of knowledge, experience and vision to achieve these adaptations. It took many more people to help us to record the infinite details of the Gerson treatment.

It is virtually impossible to thank by name all who were involved in the production of this book. They are the Gerson-trained physicians, the nurses and the helpers who produce the hourly juices—and of vital importance, the dedicated caregivers who carry out the daily routine needed for healing. The patients, too, are our heroes, disciplined and steady in their adherence to the therapy. It took those friends, acquaintances and family members who encouraged patients to stay on course and not to give up just because their original doctor gave them a death warrant.

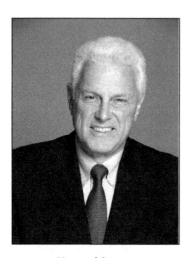
Howard Straus

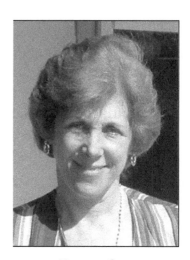
Margaret Straus

It took my son, Howard Straus, to contribute to this book with uncounted hours of research for references, ideas and suggestions, to put the information on the World Wide Web and to lecture in the United States, Canada and Asia.

It took my daughter, Margaret Straus, whose lectures, seminars, editing, articles and publicity introduced the Gerson Therapy into England, Ireland and Italy, and whose help and encouragement of patients inspired one of our most famous successes, my dear friend, Beata Bishop.

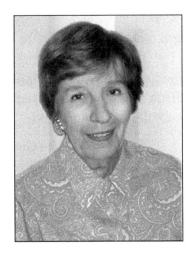

Beata Bishop

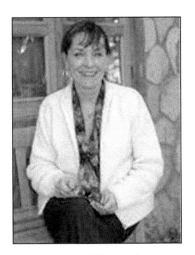

Yvonne Nienstadt

First as a dedicated patient, rewarded with a dramatic recovery, Beata Bishop introduced the Gerson Therapy into Hungary 20 years ago, where she founded the Hungarian Gerson Support Group, which now has its own residential Gerson facility, staffed by trained Gerson doctors and a Gerson therapist. In 1993, Beata helped found the Gerson Support Group UK where she remains an active member. We are very grateful to this group for allowing us to use many recipes from their publication, *Gerson Gourmet*. Other contributors to the recipe chapter include Yvonne Nienstadt, Susan DeSimone and several recovered Gerson patients.

It is virtually impossible to thank by name all who were involved in the production of this book. Here are the key players:

- President of Gerson Media & Editor in Chief: Howard Straus
- Publishing Supervisor & Design Coordinator: Sensei Bill Handel

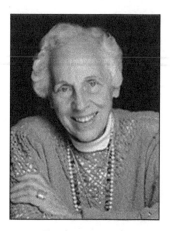

Charlotte Gerson

Many more people helped, encouraged and supported us, psychologically and often financially, to produce this project. To all the dedicated supporters continuing Dr Gerson's healing work, I devote this book with the deepest gratitude.

—Charlotte Gerson
Bonita, California
May 2011

List of Acronyms

DDT	dichloro-diphenyl-trichloroethane (pesticide)
DKP	diketopiperazine
DMARD	disease-modifying antirheumatic drug
DNA	deoxyribonucleic acid
EAFUS	"Everything" Added to Food in the United States
FDA	[U.S.] Food and Drug Administration
GE	genetically engineered
GI	gastrointestinal
GMO	genetically modified organism
GRAS	generally recognized as safe
HDL	high-density lipoprotein ("good" cholesterol)
HVO	hydrogenated vegetable oil
JAMA	*Journal of the American Medical Association*
LDL	low-density lipoprotein ("bad" cholesterol)
MCTD	mixed connective tissue disease
MSG	monosodium glutamate
NaCl	table salt, chemical composition sodium (Na) + chlorine (Cl)
NCI	[U.S.] National Cancer Institute
NIH	National Institutes of Health
NSAID	nonsteroidal anti-inflammatory drug

NPK	nitrogen, phosphorus and potassium
OTC	over-the-counter [pain-relieving drugs]
PCRM	Physicians Committee for Responsible Medicine
RA	rheumatoid arthritis
rBGH	recombinant bovine growth hormone
SAD	Standard American Diet
SLE	systemic lupus erythematosus
TEDMED	Technology & Medicine 2010 Conference (Richard Saul Wurman, Founder; Marc Hodosh, President)
USDA	U.S. Department of Agriculture

Introduction

D r. Max Gerson discovered early in his career that the body will heal when supplied with the right nutrients, and when it is cleared of poisonous substances. When he was newly settled in his practice in Bielefeld, Germany, in the mid-1920s, other doctors in the city were annoyed because he was able to help many of the patients they had not been able to treat successfully.

One such patient was Mrs. Lilly Steinhaus, in her late thirties and a mother of two children. She was suffering from rheumatoid arthritis (RA), which had frozen every joint in her body into immobility. That included her jaws, so that she had to be fed through a tube squeezed between her teeth! All her doctors were helpless.

When she was brought to Dr. Gerson's office, he used his nutritional therapy to eventually heal her completely so that she was able to function normally. She was even able to dance!

Gerson's local colleagues were angry and attacked Dr. Gerson. Their amusing premise was to claim that he cured this patient in order to generate publicity!

Dr. Gerson also found that virtually all other degenerative, chronic diseases responded positively to vegetarian, salt-free nutrition, not only rheumatoid diseases but life-threatening ones, including cancer. He felt that cancer was caused by the most severe damage to the body's defenses and, since he was able to positively influence even advanced malignancies, he was convinced that other chronic diseases would respond even more easily.

In the course of research for the present volume, we found that every rheumatoid, bone, joint and collagen disease is categorized as "incurable," with unknown etiology (cause). In fact, recent books on the subject completely avoid all discussion of etiology! All that medical science can do with these ailments is to alleviate some of the worst pain. Those very diseases have been cured quite readily with Gerson's nutritional therapy for over 80 years.

His unusual approach to medical treatment resulted in continued attacks from the orthodox medical world. In 1949, the *Journal of the American Medical Association (JAMA)* published Gerson's work with his name and curriculum vitae under the heading "Frauds and Fables."[1] It took decades, much work and many recovered patients to change the tone of a significant group of conventional medical doctors.

On Nov. 7–11, 2010, in San Diego, California, at the Science & Clinical Application of Integrative Holistic Medicine conference, sponsored by the Scripps Center for Integrative Medicine and The American Board of Integrative Holistic Medicine, Mark Hyman, MD, Chairman of the Institute for Functional Medicine, gave a presentation titled "Introduction to Functional Medicine–Redefining Disease; Applied Systems Medicine." Over 400 medical doctors attended the conference.

The theme and most of the debate centered on the "New Science on How to Prevent and Treat Cancer" and was essentially credited to Mark Hyman. However, all the other presenting physicians, some 60 in number—and without exception—recommended "diet and change of lifestyle along with supplements and body-mind resources over pharmaceuticals."[2]

Although Dr. Gerson had fully developed this approach over 80 years earlier, his name was not mentioned.

The "thread that ran throughout the conference was that disease is a systemic problem and we have to treat the system, not the symptom: the cause, not the disease," according to the *HuffPost Social News*,[3] which reported on the activities of the meeting. This completely redefines the whole notion of disease.

The new "functional medicine" is "the medicine of *why*, not *what*."[4] Dr. Hyman explains by saying, "Functional medicine is a systems biology approach to personalized medicine that focuses on the underlying causes of disease."[5]

The use of the term "New Science" in the phrase "New Science on How to Prevent and Treat Cancer" (and chronic diseases) is surprising. For example, there were other highly placed research leaders connected with this "New Science":

- Greg Lucier, chairman of Life Technologies, discussed how thinking about specific cancers is essentially flawed.

- Anna Barker, deputy director of the National Cancer Institute, explained how new teams of researchers are collaborating to think differently about cancer and treat it as a systemic problem.

"Surprisingly, scientific literature is abundant with evidence that diet, exercise, thoughts, feelings and environmental toxins all influence the initiation, growth and progression of cancer. **If a nutrient-poor diet full of sugar, lack of exercise, chronic stress, persistent pollutants and heavy metals can cause chronic disease, could it be that a nutrient-dense, plant-based diet, physical activity, changing thoughts and reactions to stress, and detoxification might treat the garden in which cancer grows? Treat the soil, not the plant.**"[6] [Emphasis added.]

We will have to treat chronic diseases by recognizing the cause. The "New Science" preaches, "We can enhance immune function and surveillance through dietary and lifestyle changes, as in phytonutrient therapies. We can facilitate our body's own detoxification system to promote the detoxification of poisonous compounds. We can improve hormone metabolism and reduce the damaging effects of too much insulin from our high sugar and refined carbohydrate diet."[7]

Dr. Gerson achieved all these aims and more, and recorded them in detail in his brilliant book, *A Cancer Therapy: Results of Fifty Cases*,[8] written and first published in 1958, and since translated and published in many languages around the world. Nonetheless, like all innovators, he was attacked by the reactionary forces of orthodox medicine. Only now are his ideas beginning to be called the "New Science" and credited to others.

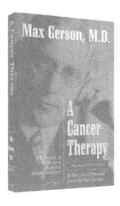

Newer publications express similar ideas, and recent films and DVDs present the information the public needs and demands: that is, how to heal their bodies rather than be cut, burned and poisoned. Enough people have witnessed and experienced the bitter futility of orthodox (drug-based) treatments. Pressure for results has built up from consumers and now, after 80 years, the orthodox medical establishment has discovered the "New Science."

REFERENCES

1. "Frauds and Fables," *JAMA*, 1949; M. Fishbein, "Cancer and the Need for Facts, Frauds and Fables," *J. Amer. Med. Ass.*, 139:2, Jan. 8, 1949, pp. 93-98.
2. Cancer Research: New Science on How to Prevent and Treat Cancer From TEDMED 2010, "Tending Your Garden: Treating the Soil in Which Cancer Grows," *HuffPost Social News*, Nov, 8, 2010.
3. M. Hyman, "Cancer Research: New Science on How to Prevent and Treat Cancer from TEDMED 2010," *HuffPost Social News* (www.huffingtonpost.com/dr-mark-hyman/cancer-new-science-on-how_b_779936.html), posted Nov. 8, 2010.
4. Ibid.
5. Ibid.
6. Ibid.
7. Ibid.
8. M. Gerson, *A Cancer Therapy: Results of Fifty Cases and The Cure of Advanced Cancer by Diet Therapy: A Summary of Thirty Years of Clinical Experimentation*, 6th ed. (San Diego, CA: Gerson Institute, 1999).

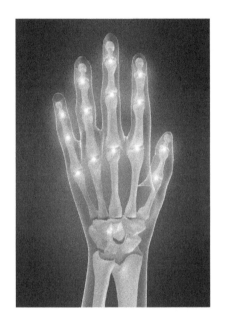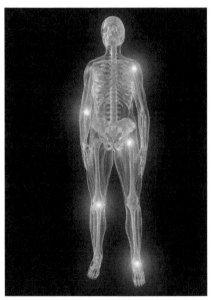

PART I

Rheumatic and Bone Diseases

CHAPTER 1

What Is Arthritis?

The term "arthritis" simply means "inflammation of the joints"[1] and is not very specific. Thus "arthritis" is actually a broad catch-all word for approximately 200 painful degenerative illnesses of your joints and the various connective tissues surrounding your joints. The most common forms of this disease are RA and osteoarthritis, with osteoarthritis making up about 95% of these two diagnoses.[2]

- RA is a disease that attacks the lining of the joints, producing symptoms from painful swelling and stiffness to large deformations and bending of the joints and bones. It is a completely different disease from osteoarthritis and mostly affects women. Allopathic medicine, unable to define a "cause" for RA, calls it an "autoimmune" disease, blaming an overactive immune system for attacking the patient's own tissue. This faulty reasoning results in treatments that involve suppressing, even killing, the immune system to keep it from doing further damage to the patient.

- Osteoarthritis breaks down the cartilage that surrounds bones and lubricates joints, causing pain and limiting mobility.

The list below includes some forms of the disease you may have heard of but may not have realized were in the arthritis family:

- Ankylosing spondylitis

- Fibromyalgia

- Gout

- Systemic lupus erythematosus (SLE)

- Scleroderma

- Osteoporosis

Although arthritis is usually associated with advancing age, it can occur in children and younger people too. In 2003, the number of Americans with "arthritis" or other chronic, rheumatoid conditions was estimated to be about 53 million, which cost the American economy about $130 billion in direct [medical] and indirect [lost wages].[3]

There are many different allopathic approaches to treating the pain associated with these diseases, including surgery (joint replacement), powerful analgesics (VIOXX), anti-inflammatories (NSAIDs), bone density drugs (e.g., Fosamax), acupuncture, weight loss and light exercise. Unfortunately however, none of these solutions will actually repair or cure damage done by the disease. Some of these remedies can be quite dangerous, and others, such as the pain-relieving drug VIOXX, have even proven fatal to significant numbers of people.[4]

Fortunately for you, the reader, all arthritic diseases yield to the Gerson Therapy. While some may heal faster and some more slowly, in time almost everyone sees a substantial benefit and very often a complete reversal of the condition.

REFERENCES

1. *Taber's Cyclopedic Medical Dictionary, 20th Edition* (Philadelphia: F. A. Davis Company, 2005), p. 173.
2. http://www.cdc.gov/arthritis/data_statistics/arthritis_related_stats.htm: The most common form of arthritis is osteoarthritis. Other common rheumatic conditions include gout, fibromyalgia and rheumatoid arthritis. An estimated 27 million adults had osteoarthritis in 2005. *Arthritis Rheum*

2008;58(1):26-35. [Data Source: NHANES] An estimated 1.5 million adults had rheumatoid arthritis in 2007.

3. http://www.cdc.gov/arthritis/data_statistics/cost.htm: The total costs attributable to arthritis and other rheumatic conditions (AORC) in the United States in 2003 was approximately $128 billion. This equaled 1.2% of the 2003 U.S. gross domestic product. $80.8 billion were direct costs (i.e., medical expenditures); $47.0 billion were indirect costs (i.e., lost earnings).

4. http://www.theweek.co.uk/us/46535/when-half-million-americans-died-and-nobody-noticed: "The recall came just days after Merck discovered that a top medical journal was about to publish a study by an FDA (Food and Drug Administration) investigator indicating that the drug in question greatly increased the risk of fatal heart attacks and strokes and had probably been responsible for at least 55,000 American deaths during the five years it had been on the market."

CHAPTER 2

Osteoarthritis

O steoarthritis is the most common form of arthritic joint disease. It affects about 95% of patients suffering from rheumatic joint problems.[1] It is defined as "a type of arthritis marked by progressive cartilage deterioration in synovial joints (joints in which the moving surfaces are lubricated by synovial fluid), that is in the vertebrae, hips and knees."[2]

The same is confirmed by Roy Altman, MD, clinical professor of rheumatology, University of California at Los Angeles, who simply states, "Osteoarthritis involves mainly fingers, hips and knees."[3]

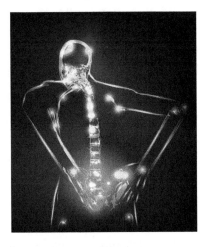

Repetitive movements, sports injuries, aging, overuse or abuse of joints are also noted as possible risk factors.[4] Obesity increases the risk for developing osteoarthritis, according to William D. Shiel, Jr., MD, FACP, FACR.[5]

The damaged joint is likely to develop lumpy outgrowths, probably due to the body's effort to mend the damage caused by loss of cartilage. Joints become painful, stiff and unresponsive.

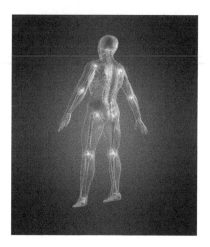

Nutrition is not mentioned as a possible cause; however, as in other conditions that are described as having an unknown cause, the Gerson Therapy has been effective in dealing with the problem. **Since hard, bony outgrowths are involved that must be dissolved, the process takes more time than healing inflammatory conditions (such as rheumatoid arthritis).** In this situation, less is reported on biochemical changes, and there are no signs of inflammation. In osteoarthritis there are fewer biochemical changes than in rheumatoid arthritis, and no signs of inflammation, bony deformities or soft tissue swellings.[6]

The real danger of this disease is the fact that it causes considerable pain, which results in patients taking over-the-counter or prescription pain-relieving drugs. These, in the case of VIOXX, for example, produce severe side effects that can be life threatening and have caused many new diseases as well as huge numbers of deaths worldwide.[7] Since the Gerson Therapy promptly clears the pain in almost all cases, patients no longer need to take these dangerous drugs.

We see many patients who present with a degree of osteoarthritis when they start on the Gerson treatment. The lumps are slowly absorbed and the disease is not further mentioned. For that reason, we have no specific "recovered patients" of that disease to illustrate.

REFERENCES

1. U.S. Department of Health & Human Services, Agency for Healthcare Research and Quality, "Rheumatoid arthritis (RA) affects one percent of the adult population. RA affects approximately 2.5 million Americans, disproportionately women." (www.qualitymeasures.ahrq.gov/content.aspx?id=8079); Health Facts, "About 42 million Americans have some form of arthritis." (http://healthfacts.wikidot.com/arthritis-osteoarthritis).

2. *Taber's Cyclopedic Medical Dictionary, 20th edition* (Philadelphia: F. A. Davis Company, 2005), p. 1541.
3. Roy Altman, MD, "How Does Osteoarthritis Differ From Rheumatoid Arthritis?" (http://abcnews.go.com/Health/PainArthritis/story?id=4561378).
4. Note 2 (*Taber's*), supra, p. 1541.
5. William C. Shiel, Jr., MD, "Diet & Osteoarthritis" (www.emedicinehealth.com/script/main/art.asp?articlekey=15021).
6. Marcus A. Krupp, MD (Clinical Professor of Medicine Emeritus, Stanford University School of Medicine, Palo Alto), ed., *Current Medical Diagnosis & Treatment* (Los Altos, CA: Lange Medical Publications, 1983), p. 501.
7. "Vioxx Side Effects" (www.drugs.com/sfx/vioxx-side-effects.html); Bill Sardi, "Just How Many Americans Did Vioxx Kill?" "Whistleblower Dr. David Graham, in testimony before the US Senate, estimated 88,000 to 139,000 Americans experienced heart attacks as a side effect from the drug, and 30 to 40 percent of these died. That would be an estimated 27,000 to 55,000 preventable deaths attributed to Vioxx." (www.lewrockwell.com/sardi/sardi53.html).

CHAPTER 3

Collagen Diseases

Rheumatoid Arthritis

In *Arthritis and Allied Conditions,* a huge collection of articles by physicians treating such disorders, this definition appears: "Rheumatoid Arthritis is a systemic connective tissue disorder of unknown etiology."[1] Much more recently, in the 2006 Merck Manual, it is also stated that "the precise cause [of rheumatoid arthritis] is unknown."[2]

Despite continued research, the notation "unknown etiology" appears in the definition of almost every single type of arthritis, in books predating 1990. Later volumes, including *Taber's Cyclopedic Dictionary* (2005), simply do not mention "etiology." This makes the disease "incurable"—if we accept that "the cure is in the cause" (see Chapter 8, "The Cure Is in the Cause," p. 43). All arthritis treatments and medications are used as symptomatic palliatives (for pain relief) and in an attempt to reduce inflammation and swelling.

Dr. Julian Whitaker writes "**Conventional doctors primarily prescribe non-steroidal anti-inflammatory drugs (NSAIDs) for arthritis.** These include ibuprofen (Motrin and Advil) and naproxen (Aleve). They have many negative side effects. **They cause 20,000 deaths a year from gastrointestinal bleeding and other complications, and in the**

long term actually worsen arthritis by accelerating cartilage destruction and blocking the body's mechanism for healing joints and regenerating cartilage."[3][Emphasis added.]

Rheumatoid arthritis is also classified as an "autoimmune" disease[4] and is often treated with methotrexate. This is still more toxic than other drugs and, in higher doses, is used as a chemotherapy drug in cancer treatments. It helps to relieve pain at the start, so patients are encouraged to take it; however, its analgesic effect weakens over time and, in a few months, the pain relief stops and only the severe side effects remain. "DMARDs [disease-modifying antirheumatic drugs] such as Methotrexate are the drugs given to more than 80% of patients treated."[5]

Another drug, in the same class as VIOXX, a so-called COX-2 inhibitor, is Celebrex, prescribed for pain relief. This drug also has extremely severe side effects such as gastrointestinal bleeding, ulceration and perforation of the stomach and intestines and kidney damage.[6]

Rheumatoid arthritis causes serious swelling of joints, mainly in fingers, toes, wrists and knees, with eventual destruction of the affected joints. It is painful and inhibits mobility and ability to work. It is more common in premenopausal women than in men by a factor of 2:1.[7] It eventually causes deformity of joints, inability to walk and possible total incapacitation due to deformity of the hands.

Numerous factors are assumed to increase susceptibility to rheumatoid arthritis including heredity (see Chapter 9, "Breakdown of the Body's Defenses," p. 53); loss of female sex hormone (menopause) and environmental factors, which are still questioned.[8] Not surprisingly, fibromyalgia (generalized bone pain) is found in a substantial number of rheumatoid arthritis patients.[9]

Fortunately, all the above problems—swelling, joint damage, pain and even serious deformity—have been eliminated with the Gerson Therapy. Cartilage reforms and fingers straighten out! The amount of time required to fully recover depends on the duration of the disease prior to the Gerson Therapy and on the amount of damage caused by the side effects of prescribed drugs.

Case History #1

"Almost 20 years ago, the Gerson Therapy brought our daughter, Susan A., back out of helpless, bedridden rheumatoid arthritis to a reasonably normal life," her father writes. "She is even horseback riding now. As for my own well-being over these past 20 years, **I have been doing a daily coffee enema and a limited Gerson natural food program. The results: No sickness, no disease, and I am still working full time as a consulting engineer at age 74.**" [Emphasis added.]

Case History #2

Penny M. had suffered from rheumatoid arthritis and was in a deplorable state. She was mostly bedfast and in severe pain. She admitted that during the previous three months, she had daily prayed for death. After she started the Gerson Therapy, the pain abated, her swellings were absorbed and she is presently (16 years later) in perfectly normal health and activity. She remains well, totally recovered and happy to be alive!

Lupus Erythematosus

In *Arthritis and Allied Conditions*, "lupus erythematosus" is described as "a disease of unknown etiology."[10] The etiology of MCTD [mixed connective tissue disease] ... is "unknown."[11] "Progressive systemic sclerosis (scleroderma)" is said to have "obscure etiology."[12] However, in the last case, there is an additional note: This disease is progressive, severe and can advance to being fatal.

These disorders appear to have in common widespread immunologic and inflammatory alterations. For our purposes, it is important to note that most of them are accompanied by "... nephritis [kidney inflammation] and alterations of many connective tissues with scarring, hyperplasia or distortions. ... Although the connective tissue disorders are regarded as acquired diseases, the underlying causes cannot be determined .. Heredity, infection, or other environmental antigen, immunoglobulin deficiency ... drug allergy ... or some combination of all of these factors appear to play varying undefined roles."[13]

Systemic Lupus Erythematosus

SLE is an inflammatory disorder that may affect multiple organ systems. Women are mainly affected. The clinical course may vary from a mild episodic disorder to a rapidly fulminating fatal illness.[14]

Joint symptoms occur in over 90% of patients and are often the earliest manifestation of the disease.[15] "There are many other symptoms, however the one with which we are mainly concerned is that several forms of renal disease are observed."[16] Proliferative glomerulonephritis (kidney inflammation) is the major threat to the life of patients suffering from SLE.[17]

The symptoms are treated with various drugs and can be suppressed temporarily but not healed. The skin eruptions may be treated with a local administration of corticosteroids. In patients with a mild form of lupus, a period of normalcy may be observed. The most serious complication, in the aggressive type of this disease, is the progressive renal (kidney) disease followed by central nervous system involvement.[18]

Early symptoms of lupus erythematosus usually include severe fatigue. It also progresses to skin rashes, fever and joint discomfort. The rash may appear in any part of the body but is frequently seen in the face, on both sides of the nose. It is therefore referred to as the "butterfly rash." In about 85% of the patients, there is also weight loss. Prednisone is used as a treatment. It causes the patients to feel better; however, in acute cases, the disease readily progresses and involves various organs to the point of death.[19]

Lupus erythematosus is studied extensively in order to ascertain if it has a possible genetic cause and/or is being influenced by environmental factors. Arthritic problems without deformity are also seen with pain on movement, tenderness and soft tissue swelling.[20]

One note seems to point in the direction of "cause." In *Arthritis and Allied Conditions,* a lengthy table has a notation that some 25% of patients show a "profuse proteinuria, greater than 3.5 g per day."[21] **("Proteinuria" is the excretion of protein by the kidneys, which** should be 0.) This indicates severe kidney damage and, more interestingly, the fact that the body is overloaded with proteins!

All of these problems yield readily to the Gerson Therapy, which is free of animal proteins, so that kidney damage can be cleared and the immune system can function normally.

Case History

"Avrill had (I can use the past tense now) been so ill for about 25 years with lupus that I felt she would never experience anything in life except pain and misery," her husband wrote. "Twenty odd years on prednisone and NSAIDS have not done her immune system much good. I think it was about six years ago that we were told about the Gerson Therapy. Avrill was so sick at the time; I thought she would die. The doctors had her on high doses of morphine to control the agonizing pain, not to mention the 50 to 80 mg of prednisone a day, as well as an array of NSAIDs. In the beginning, Avrill was not that keen to do the Gerson Therapy, but I think she finally came to the conclusion that she had little choice. The doctors had told her that there was nothing more that they could do for her.

"Avrill's recovery has been steady and spectacular. She is finally completely drug free. She still has one coffee enema each day and is healthier now, at 48 years of age, than she has been all her life. Over the last 12 months, she has had two operations to try to straighten her fingers. The damage was caused to the tendons by a cocktail of drugs she had taken over the years. Physically, she is in excellent condition. She looks much younger than her age and is able to do almost anything. She actively gardens, uses a petrol [gasoline]-powered brush cutter, shifts rocks into garden borders, collects wood, etc. Not bad for someone who, a few years ago, could not comb her own hair or lift a dinner plate from the table! I am very proud of her."

Avrill's husband adds another significant detail to her story. It seems that, during her treatment, she "cheated" several times. "In the early days, if she strayed off her diet and had fish 'n' chips or a hamburger, it usually meant a trip to the hospital within 48 hours for a morphine needle!" Avrill's husband feels that this does not belong in a recovered patient report; on the contrary, we are very much aware that, at times, patients will stray from the straight and narrow. The dramatic results, in her case, should be a warning to other "cheaters."

"Avrill has come a long way since then," her husband continues. "I was talking to her tonight and she was commenting on how quickly the surgery incisions on her hands had completely healed without so much as a scar. In the old days, a cut or scratch would take weeks or months to heal, and usually after several infections. Thanks to the Gerson Therapy and what we have learned from your books and newsletters, Avrill has, for the first time in her life, a working immune system."

Please note that lupus is supposed to be an "autoimmune disease" with the immune system working overtime!

Lupus, Fibromyalgia and Myelofibrosis

It is difficult to convince doctors that all chronic degenerative diseases are basically caused by two major problems: toxicity and nutritional deficiency. For that reason, when we can help the patient with hyperalimentation (i.e., feeding the deficient patient with the correct, living organic nutrients) as well as detoxification, it is perfectly possible to cure most of the so-called "incurable" diseases.

One of these, a relatively rare condition, is called "myelofibrosis," which is "a myeloproliferative disorder marked by the overproduction of a single stem cell clone and reactive bone marrow fibrosis."[22] However, in this case, the disease overlaps with others, including lupus and fibromyalgia.

Case History

By the time Bob O. was 58 years old, he had suffered for many years from constant bone pain. This started on his return from Vietnam in 1970, after he had been exposed to Agent Orange and other toxic materials.

For many years, during the 80s and 90s, he only took aspirin. However, when he reported to the U.S. Department of Veterans Affairs hospital, he was prescribed 3,000 mg per day of ibuprofen for pain relief. He actually took this huge amount for one to two years until it finally severely damaged his stomach. Meanwhile, he was also diagnosed with lupus and, some time later, with fibromyalgia. His skin was also sick: it blistered, scabbed, flaked and was scaly.

He finally stopped taking ibuprofen and creams. In spite of his damaged stomach, constant pain and damaged skin, he never stopped working. He had joined the carpenter's union and worked in carpentry, a very toxic occupation with its solvents, glues containing formaldehyde and chemically treated wood.

In 1996, he quit carpentry and went into pipe welding—no less toxic—till September 2006, all this time suffering with "whole body pain" where all his joints and bones were constantly hurting.

Finally, one day, as he was going to bed, he noted that there was a large bump on his left side. This sent him to a doctor, who found that Bob's spleen was hugely swollen. While he looked at it, the doctor did nothing!

Shortly after that, Bob "crashed." He was unable to get up and work because he was in so much pain. The swelling in his spleen had become so severe that it extended from his pelvis to his rib cage. His wife, Judy, says that he looked grey. Of course, he was severely anemic since his bone marrow, turned largely into scar tissue, was unable to produce red blood cells!

He was finally diagnosed adequately by a doctor in a cancer hospital in Columbia, Missouri, who did a bone marrow biopsy. The Ellis Fischel Hospital, a part of the University of Missouri complex, specializes in cancer. On recognizing and reconfirming that Bob was suffering from myelofibrosis, he suggested a drug called thalidomide, which had a less than 30% chance of reducing the swelling of the spleen within six months but which also had very severe side effects. Bob declined to take the drug.

In that case, the doctor said, there was nothing he could do, and suggested that Bob go home and get his affairs in order. Nevertheless, he also suggested that Bob return for another check-up in three months. When Bob did come back, the doctor was amazed that he was still alive!

At last, Bob O. heard of the Gerson Caregiver training and attended the December 2006 session in San Diego. **Amazingly, from almost the first enema Bob ever took, after overcoming his natural resistance to such a procedure, he was virtually free of pain—for the first time in 30 years!**

While Bob had started on the Gerson Therapy a little earlier on his own, he went to the Mexican Gerson hospital. Now, a little over a year later, he feels very well. He has *no pain*, and Dr. M., who is a doctor at the Gerson Mexican hospital, tells him that his blood test is almost entirely normal. His bone marrow is miraculously producing the needed red and white cells again. Bob states that his spleen is down by about 50% and there is still a ways to go.

Mixed Collagen Disease

From the name, we understand that this is a disease of "overlapping features" of the other connective tissue diseases, including SLE, scleroderma and myositis, as well as Raynaud's disease[23] (see above).

Patients also usually have arthritis, with taut and thickened skin. In a study that lasted six years, 4% of patients died.[24] Longer term follow-up studies showed that many patients subsequently developed scleroderma.[25] With less serious renal and central nervous system disease, patients respond to low doses of corticosteroids. Mild disease is often controlled with NSAIDs.[26]

All the connective tissue diseases described above are totally curable by the Gerson Therapy with its usual *detoxifying and rebuilding* effect.

Case History

Born in 1964, Anne was an inveterate distance runner, even in high school. At the age of 38, in 2001, she first noticed swelling in her hands that didn't abate at night or in a few days. She also had some pain and difficulty closing her hands normally. That is when she consulted her doctor.

A nurse practitioner attended her and ran a lot of tests, which showed positive for lupus. Anne then consulted a rheumatologist, who confirmed "mixed connective tissue disease," which includes lupus, rheumatoid arthritis and scleroderma.

The doctor prescribed plaquinel, steroids and methotrexate (a chemotherapy drug prescribed for patients assumed to suffer from autoimmune disease, since it severely depresses the immune system). Anne took those drugs for one year but didn't feel any better; however, admittedly, she did not feel worse. She had to quit her job, lost a good deal of hair and had a puffed face. She refused to take these drugs any longer and for one additional year took nothing.

Anne did a lot of research and read as much as she could find. During that year, she found the natural healing approach of George Malkmus[27] and started juicing. She felt better and the disease didn't seem to progress.

In September 2002, she had a severe lupus attack. She decided to go to the Mayo Clinic, even though it had a long waiting list. She arrived in February 2005. There, all tests were done again and the rheumatologist stated that she now had scleroderma, polymyelitis with weak muscles and Raynaud's disease.

He realized that Anne would resist drug treatments, so he pressured her by stating—in her husband's presence—that, without drugs, she would be in a wheelchair within six months.

The rheumatologist then prescribed a drug—an immune suppressant, which is usually given to patients who receive liver transplants. The drug was described to her as a "low-grade, fever-type aspirin." After taking this drug, Anne went into shock and landed in intensive care for two weeks where she almost died.

Anne was given many more drugs but doesn't know exactly what they were since she was "out of it." When she finally recovered from this treatment, she started to research the drug this doctor had given her and found out that it causes liver cancer. It also caused her to gain 30 pounds during those two weeks. Then they gave her another drug, which apparently drained this accumulation.

Her regular doctor at home actually suggested that she try the Gerson Therapy. She found *A Cancer Therapy: Results of Fifty Cases*,[28] then checked the recovered patient list given to her by the Gerson Institute. Encouraged and hopeful, she came to the Mexican Gerson hospital in May 2005.

In February 2007, Anne wrote to her Gerson doctor, "I am doing wonderfully!" On her two-year Gerson anniversary, she visited the Mexican Gerson clinic and showed herself to the other patients, who are always very happy to meet recovered patients and who are encouraged by seeing them well and active.

Scleroderma

"Scleroderma" is a systemic sclerosis, a chronic disorder characterized by diffuse fibrosis (scarring) of the skin and internal organs and classified with the connective tissue diseases. Its cause is unknown.[29] Women are affected two to three times as frequently as men.[30]

This disorder takes several forms. Some scarring, called "morphea," is formed on the skin. This is defined as "a chronic manifestation of progressive systemic sclerosis in which the skin is taut, firm and edematous, limiting movement."[31]

Scleroderma can appear as a relatively benign, slowly progressive disorder, often showing up as Raynaud's phenomenon[32] (restriction of blood flow to the extremities, sometimes causing numbness and atrophy of the skin; cause unknown).[33]

In some patients, the disease takes a different form and other organs are involved. Some cases involve an overlapping syndrome called "mixed connective tissue disease."[34] Still another group may show systemic sclerosis that is rapidly progressive; its course, due to the involvement of major viscera, may lead to death within a few years.[35] The disease can also affect the intestines and cause scarring, reduced lung capacity and heart failure.[36]

In this pathology, the Gerson Therapy has also proved very effective.

REFERENCES

1. Daniel J. McCarty, MD, ed., *Arthritis and Allied Conditions: A Textbook of Rheumatology, Ninth Edition* (Philadelphia: Lea & Febiger, 1979), p. 78.
2. "Rheumatoid Arthritis (RA)" (www.merckmanuals.com/professional/sec04/ch034/ch034b.html).
3. J. Whitaker, MD, *Dr. Whitaker's Unabridged Dictionary of Drug Alternatives and Non-surgical Solutions* (Potomac, MD: Healthy Directions, LLC, 2007), p. 6.
4. Raashid Luqmani, Theodore Pincus and Maarten Boers, eds., *Rheumatoid Arthritis* (Oxford: Oxford University Press, Oxford Rheumatology Library, 2010), p. 11.
5. Ibid., p. 49.
6. Ibid., p. 7.
7. T. K. Kvien, A. Glennas, et al., "The prevalence and severity of rheumatoid arthritis in Oslo," *Scand J Rheumatol,* 1997;26:412-18; T. K. Kvien, T. Uhlig, et al., "Epidemiological aspects of rheumatoid arthritis: the sex ratio," *Ann N Y Acad Sci,* 2006;1069:212-22.
8. Note 4 (Luqmani, et al.), supra, p. 8.
9. Ibid., p. 21.
10. Note 1 (McCarty), supra, p. 691.
11. Ibid., p. 740.
12. Ibid., p. 762.
13. Marcus A. Krupp, MD (Clinical Professor of Medicine Emeritus, Stanford University School of Medicine, Palo Alto), ed., *Current Medical Diagnosis & Treatment* (Los Altos, CA: Lange Medical Publications, 1983), p. 485.
14. Ibid., p. 490.
15. Ibid., p. 491.
16. Ibid.

17. Ibid.

18. Ibid., p. 492.

19. Note 1 (McCarty), supra, p. 692.

20. Ibid., p. 697.

21. Ibid.

22. *Taber's Cyclopedic Medical Dictionary, 20th edition* (Philadelphia: F. A. Davis Company, 2005), p. 1414.

23. Note 13 (Krupp), supra, p. 494.

24. Ibid.

25. Ibid.

26. Ibid.

27. For more information about Rev. George Malkmus Lit. D., see http://cpbooks.christianpost.com/Rev-George-Malkmus-Lit-D-/389).

28. M. Gerson, *A Cancer Therapy: Results of Fifty Cases and The Cure of Advanced Cancer by Diet Therapy: A Summary of Thirty Years of Clinical Experimentation*, 6th ed. (San Diego, CA: Gerson Institute, 1999).

29. Note 13 (Krupp), supra, p. 493.

30. Ibid.

31. Note 22 (*Taber's*), supra, p. 1957.

32. Note 13 (Krupp), supra, p. 493.

33. Note 22 (*Taber's*), supra, p. 1957.

34. Note 13 (Krupp), supra, p. 493.

35. Ibid.

36. Ibid.

CHAPTER 4

Ankylosing Spondylitis

The ailment "ankylosing spondylitis" starts with chronic backaches and generally affects young males. It progresses to a limitation of back motion and of chest expansion. Later, it becomes indistinguishable from rheumatoid arthritis. The back pain may radiate down the thighs and gradually stiffen the spine, often leading to fusion of the vertebrae. The preponderance in males is approximately 10:1.[1]

A major difference between ankylosing spondylitis and rheumatoid arthritis is that the former rarely involves the small joints of the hands and feet, nor does it produce subcutaneous (below-the-skin) nodules. In some individuals, fluoride poisoning may be present.[2] Once again, it is noted that "the etiology of this disease is unknown."[3] Ankylosing spondylitis is described as "a chronic progressive inflammatory disorder."[4] The major form of treatment is the use of NSAIDs. Spontaneous remissions and relapses are common.[5]

As in virtually all other rheumatoid diseases, there is no cure with orthodox treatments, yet almost all of them are totally curable with the Gerson Therapy.

Case History #1

At a convention in Phoenix, Arizona, a gentleman from the audience came up to the podium and testified about his recovery using the Gerson Therapy. He confided that he had been suffering from ankylosing spondylitis some 20 years ago. His spine was virtually paralyzed and he was on 100% disability. At the time, he was unable to close his hand or raise his arm, but showed the audience how he could now raise his arm normally. He had heard one of the Gerson lectures at a Chicago health convention many years before and had done the Gerson Therapy at home, on his own, for two years. He ran—covering 10,000 miles over the last 20 years—and swam regularly and was in excellent condition. He stated that he had not spent a penny on doctors or drugs during those previous 20 years, not even for aspirin. He had had no headaches or colds.

Case History #2

We received a letter from a gentleman who wrote the following: "I was diagnosed with pneumonia and emphysema, as well as lymphoma (and more). In April, I will have been on the Gerson Therapy for two years. All degenerative diseases have gone: glaucoma, Reiters Syndrome, ankylosing spondylitis, arrhythmia and emphysema. All the lymphoma tumors are gone or vastly reduced. **For the first time in 30 years I am completely pain free.**" [Emphasis added.]

Case History #3

William Goerdes was brought into Dr. Gerson's office on a stretcher. He was in his early forties; however, his spine was totally paralyzed with ankylosing spondylitis. He had worked in the construction business and was obviously completely disabled.

On the Gerson Therapy, his pain was relieved and he started to move. It took a year before he was able to get up and walk. **As it turns out, the family did not have an electric juice extractor, so the wife ground up the vegetables, then pressed them through a tight cloth by hand to make juice!** Within a few years, he was completely cured to the point where, at age 50, he was able to go back to heavy iron work in the construction business. He remained well and able to walk totally erect for the rest of his life.

His son, in his early twenties, also contracted ankylosing spondylitis, pointing to the possibility that the tendency to develop this disease is genetic. He healed himself and, according to his grandmother, is presently in good health.

Much later, when William was 82 years old, his wife passed away. At that time, while he continued to be in excellent health, he started to date actively and loved to dance. He only complained that his girlfriends always became ill and died. We suggested that he pick younger ones. He answered that he had done that but those, too, died! He lived to the age of 97, in good physical and mental health, and died of pneumonia.

REFERENCES

1. Marcus A. Krupp, MD (Clinical Professor of Medicine Emeritus, Stanford University School of Medicine, Palo Alto), ed., *Current Medical Diagnosis & Treatment* (Los Altos, CA: Lange Medical Publications, 1983), p. 98.
2. Ibid.
3. Daniel J. McCarty, MD, ed., *Arthritis and Allied Conditions: A Textbook of Rheumatology, Ninth Edition* (Philadelphia: Lea & Febiger, 1979), p. 620.
4. *Taber's Cyclopedic Medical Dictionary, 20th edition* (Philadelphia: F. A. Davis Company, 2005), p. 2053.
5. Note 1 (Krupp), supra, p. 499.

CHAPTER 5

Gout

The disease "gout" is described as a metabolic disease and, in about 50% of cases, first presents with severe pain in the midjoint of the big toe.[1] There are many asymptomatic periods between acute attacks.[2] As we have pointed out, many of the rheumatic diseases are characterized by kidney damage. **Gout is usually caused by the body's overproduction or underexcretion of uric acid, a process normally handled by the kidneys.** Aside from kidney disease, drugs and lead poisoning have also been associated with gout.[3]

Uric acid and kidney stones, along with kidney dysfunction, are present in 10% to 20% of patients with gouty arthritis.[4] Patients with gout also have an increased incidence of hypertension, renal diseases and diabetes mellitus.[5] "However these relationships are not well understood."[6]

Gout responds very well to the drug colchicine; however, patients manifest considerable hyperuricemia (excessive amount of uric acid in the blood),[7] which causes crystal formation. The crystals lodge especially in the joints of the big toe and produce considerable pain. However, they are also found in subcutaneous tissue, bone, cartilage, joints and other tissues. Ninety-five percent of gout occurs in males.[8]

The presence of gout points seriously to an overconsumption of animal proteins. This is further confirmed by the following findings: Nephrosclerosis (hardening of the connective tissues of the kidneys)[9] with renal dysfunction is common.[10] **This is another reason why the Gerson Therapy is so effective in overcoming gout.**

"As the symptoms of an attack progress the pain becomes intense. The involved joints are swollen and exquisitely tender and the overlying skin tense, warm and dusky red. Fever, headache, malaise, anorexia [loss of appetite[11]] and tachycardia [an abnormally high heart rate, exceeding 100 beats per minute in adults[12]] are common. Asymptomatic periods of months or more, commonly follow the initial acute attack. Later gouty arthritis may become chronic with symptoms of progressive functional loss and disability. Hypertension, renal stones and renal failure may be associated with gouty arthritis."[13]

Recovered Patient Story

A patient arrived at the Gerson Therapy clinic in Mexico with several serious problems. He was in his late 30s, married and had two children.

His father had been a Gerson patient several years earlier, suffering from advanced pancreatic cancer as well as heart disease. He had been treated previously with bypass surgery but, on the Gerson treatment, recovered completely from his pancreatic cancer.

His son, the new patient, was grossly overweight. He had uncontrollable diabetes with a blood sugar level above 250, which could not be reduced with drugs. Aside from his morbid obesity, he was also suffering from gout and was on daily medication to keep it under control. He stated that, if he skipped his gout medication for only one day, he would suffer a painful gout attack.

In such cases, it is often necessary for Gerson doctors to wean patients off the medications they are using. This was done with his heart drugs. However, despite warnings, the gout medication was stopped "cold turkey." **To his own great surprise, on the purely vegetarian Gerson diet, he never had another attack!**

Along with his salt-free vegetarian meals, he was also given platters of "Gerson snacks" served in his room should he get hungry. These contained cherry tomatoes, green pepper strips, carrot sticks, radishes and green onions. He reported that, with the regular juices, he was never hungry. He lost over 100 pounds in six weeks, felt great and was close to normal at 210 pounds with his 6'3" height. His diabetes had also disappeared without further medication.

Important note: As we have specifically noted with a number of other patients, arthritic problems are often associated with kidney dysfunction. It is important to understand that the kidneys are involved, among other functions, in excreting the end products of (animal) protein digestion.[14] For that reason, with poor kidney function, those products are not adequately excreted and cause a great deal of arthritic pain and inflammation.

REFERENCES

1. Marcus A. Krupp, MD (Clinical Professor of Medicine Emeritus, Stanford University School of Medicine, Palo Alto), ed., *Current Medical Diagnosis & Treatment* (Los Altos, CA: Lange Medical Publications, 1983), p. 504.
2. Ibid.
3. Ibid.
4. Ibid., p. 505.
5. Ibid., p. 506.
6. Ibid.
7. *Taber's Cyclopedic Medical Dictionary, 20th edition* (Philadelphia: F. A. Davis Company, 2005), p. 1045.
8. Note 1 (Krupp), supra.
9. Note 7 (*Taber's*), supra, p. 1441.
10. Note 1 (Krupp), supra, p. 505.
11. Note 7 (*Taber's*), supra, p. 127.
12. Ibid., p. 2137.
13. Note 1 (Krupp), supra, p. 505.
14. Ibid., p. 531.

CHAPTER 6

Fibromyalgia

F ibromyalgia is a new disease. In dictionaries, medical texts and arthritis books that predate 1990, you will not find the term. It is now described as **"a chronic and frequently difficult to manage pain in muscles and soft tissues surrounding joints."**[1] [Emphasis added.] Treatment approaches include reassurance, physical therapy, with the objective of restoring normal neuromuscular function, cardiovascular fitness and appropriate medications for sleep disturbances. Drugs include topical capsacin, oral anti-inflammatories, antidepressants and/ or narcotic analgesics.[2]

There is no mention of prognosis, course of the disease, or possible improvement.

Case History

Here is a patient's own story, titled "Seven Years of Fibromyalgia":

"At the age of 16, I felt as if I were 90. I went from being a gymnast, musician and honor student, to a lethargic medical mess. After a week-long hospital stay for an abscessed tonsil, I did not feel well again for seven years. I began to ache and drag, always waiting to regain the corporal vigor I once enjoyed.

"After frequent complaints to my mother of how my body felt sore, achy, tired and weak, she took me to see our family doctor. He referred me to a pediatric rheumatologist at Loma Linda Children's Hospital in Loma Linda, California. I remember being quite optimistic and confident that the doctors there would be able to help me relieve my pain.

"I showed them where it hurt and explained what it felt like. I was tested for various diseases and a diagnosis was given. What causes this fibromyalgia, and how do I get rid of it? These are the obvious next questions after one is diagnosed with any illness.

"My trusted physician, Dr. Roberts, explained that this was a 'new' condition, that it was unusual but not unheard of in a person of my age, and that there was intense research being done, but there is no cure. He said I could grow out of it, that it was not a degenerative disease, some get better, some get worse. I was crushed by the thought of trudging through life in pain, pretending as if all was well. It became necessary to pretend I felt better than I did. I couldn't bear to watch my mother cry anymore because she felt so helpless. She felt my pain as did the rest of my family.

"When was this nightmare going to end? I don't remember the first drug I was prescribed, or the fifth, but I do remember the last. My appointments consisted of a few questions about how I was feeling, and if the prescribed medication was doing the trick. The answer was always no and the treatment was adjusted accordingly. Different drug or different doses, I was allowed to choose. I chose to stop taking liver-toxic, mind-numbing drugs.

"This decision was made after I got into the car in my pink fuzzy slippers, driving around, not knowing where or why I was going. I was taking Elivel, an antidepressant. Antidepressants in certain doses are often given to patients suffering from fibromyalgia. After I informed Dr. Roberts that I would no longer be testing any more chemical concoctions, he told me I was depressed. I began to cry in the doctor's office and he asked my mother to leave the room. He asked if there was something I wanted to say in confidence to him.

"I told him I was not depressed; I was just in constant pain. I was always tired and sluggish. I had to literally roll out of bed and drag myself to school, achy and miserable.

"'What can I do?' I asked him. 'If you cannot help me, then who can?'" [Emphasis added.]

"I left that day frustrated and longing for answers. That doctor never once asked about what I was eating or what my bowel movements were like. **I knew it would be my responsibility to take my health into my own hands, stomach and every other part I owned.** I decided to experiment on myself and pay close attention to what I ate and how I felt afterwards. I vowed to finish medical school, my lifelong dream, and find a cure for the ever-present fibromyalgia. **I initially eliminated fast food and soda. I did feel better but still not well.** [Emphasis added.]

"After trudging through college and work, in agony for seven years, I was able to heal, thanks to Dr. Max Gerson. My older sister called one day to ask if I needed a job. The timing was perfect. I did need a job, and Gerson.

"All I knew at first about my sister's job was that she made juice for some guy. A whole new world of living: fresh, organic, nutritious foods came to my attention. The kitchen was regarded as the nurse's station and the food as medicine. My boss, Tim, encouraged me to drink juice, eat the living food, and even sent me on my maiden voyage (with coffee?) to the "healing room" (also known as the bathroom).

"The almost immediate change in my physical health was astounding. For the first time, I had no pain. After seven years of feeling awful, this was a foreign concept. My skin, which had become riddled with acne, began to clear. Even the old scars started to fade. My mental clarity, energy and mood returned.

"There was and is a cure for fibromyalgia and every other chronic degenerative disease. As an individual who has always been fascinated with the human body's infinitely intricate inner workings, **I am forever grateful to Dr. Max Gerson for his genius and courage. I am forever grateful to Charlotte Gerson and all others who perpetuate his message.** [Emphasis added.]

"The basic components of all things are essentially the same. Electrically charged atoms bump into one another, combining, repelling and making up not only our bodies but every other substance in the entire universe.

The body is constructed from the simplest of elements and arranged into endlessly complex systems that must be nurtured and not just fed. Each individual must claim responsibility for their own construction or demise.

"I am just one living example of the potent effectiveness of respecting the intimate relationship between our internal and external metabolism. **Organic juice, food and coffee enemas saved my life. I am so happy to be alive.**" [Emphasis added.]

REFERENCES

1. *Taber's Cyclopedic Medical Dictionary, 20th edition* (Philadelphia: F. A. Davis Company, 2005), p. 797.
2. Ibid.

CHAPTER 7

Osteoporosis

I f you search the Internet and look up "osteoporosis," you'll find this: **"Osteoporosis is the most commonly seen metabolic bone disease in the USA."**[1] [Emphasis added.] It is defined as "a condition common in older patients, and particularly women, that is characterized by the thinning of bone tissue and loss of bone density over time.[2] The article further states: "The leading causes of osteoporosis are a drop in estrogen in women at the time of menopause and a drop in testosterone in men. The disease occurs in women in their 50s and in men around the age of 70. It is more common in men who smoke!"[3]

A number of books note the relationship between excess (animal) protein consumption and osteoporosis.[4]

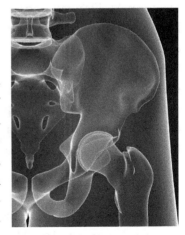

A more recent development occurred when the Physicians Committee for Responsible Medicine (PCRM) lodged a complaint in January 1997 with the Federal Trade Commission in Washington, DC, about a new advertising campaign sponsored by the National Fluid Milk Processor Promotion Board, saying "with calcium galore [milk] is one of the best things around."[5] At that time, the ads featured the new "celebrity milk mustache."

The PCRM says that "increasing milk consumption is one of the weakest possible strategies for protecting the bones and to suggest otherwise is dangerously misleading."[6] [Emphasis added.] On the contrary, physicians in the above group found that "Countries with high calcium intake typically have much higher fracture rates compared to countries with lower calcium intakes."[7]

More importantly, this group is very much aware and states that "Dietary and lifestyle factors that encourage the loss of bone calcium include: animal protein, sodium, (salt), caffeine, phosphorus, tobacco and a sedentary lifestyle. For example, eliminating meat from the diet was found in one study to cut urinary calcium losses in half. Cutting sodium intake in half can reduce calcium requirements by 160 milligrams per day. **Avoiding tobacco has demonstrable effectiveness: smokers have 10% weaker bones compared to non-smokers."[8]** [Emphasis added.]

"In every study the same correspondence was found: the more protein that is taken in, the more calcium is lost."[9] [Emphasis added.]

"Summarizing the medical research on osteoporosis, one of the nation's leading medical authorities on dietary associations with disease, Dr. John McDougall, says: '**I would like to emphasize that the calcium-losing effect of [animal] protein on the human body is not an area of controversy in scientific circles. The many studies performed during the past fifty-five years consistently show that the most important dietary change that we can make if we want to create a positive calcium balance that will keep our bones solid is to decrease the amount of proteins we eat each day.** The important change is not to increase the amount of calcium we take in.'"[10] [Emphasis added.]

John Robbins reports that he found no basis at all for the Dairy Council's viewpoint recommending that American women should take in 1,200 mg of calcium daily. "African Bantu Women take in only 350 mg of calcium per day. They bear (an average of) nine children during their lifetime and breast feed them for two years. They never have calcium deficiency, seldom break a bone, rarely lose a tooth. They are on a low protein diet that doesn't kick the calcium out of the body. In our country, those who can afford it, are eating 20% of their total calories in protein, which guarantees a negative mineral balance, not only of calcium, but of magnesium, zinc and iron. It's all directly related to the amount of protein you eat."[11]

The real danger of osteoporosis is not only the negative calcium and mineral balance but the drugs that are prescribed by physicians to their patients to supposedly maintain healthy bones. They have never promised to rebuild bones, and they present extremely damaging side effects.

Serious Dangers from Fosamax, Actonel and Boniva "Bone-Building Drugs"

This report appeared in the British Medical Journal (January 2008),[12] but it is extremely timely because of the continuing powerful advertising campaign for these dangerous drugs.

Fosamax, Actonel and Boniva belong in the group of "bisphosphonate" drugs. Here's how they function: Healthy bones maintain their strength from a continual process of bone breakdown and bone rebuilding. "Osteoclasts" are the cells that break down bone, and "osteoblasts" are the cells that rebuild it.

Fosamax and similar drugs poison osteoclasts, permanently killing them and the normal bone-repair process is halted! So, your bones will indeed get denser; however, denser bones are not stronger bones, which is the part they don't tell you. In fact, bones eventually become older, *weaker and more prone to fracture!*

Merck (the manufacturer) tried to hide the fact that Fosamax is causing jawbone death,[13] a disease now known to oral surgeons as bisphosphonate-associated osteonecrosis (death of the jaw) or "phossy jaw," a nasty side effect of Fosamax and similar drugs. Essentially, the condition causes your jawbone to rot and decay—quite ironic, considering these drugs are taken by people hoping to strengthen their bones.

In addition, bisphosphonates have also been associated with:

- Serious eye inflammation and possible blindness
- Liver damage
- Atrial fibrillation (heart irregularity)
- Increased risk of ulcers
- Esophageal cancer
- Renal failure (kidney damage)

Merck did not disclose these problems or the damage done by VIOXX, which killed many thousands.[14] It was supposed to be only for pain control.

Further problems with Fosamax, Actonel and Boniva are causing serious trouble because they *stay in the bone indefinitely and disrupt the normal bone regeneration process!* [15] The condition cannot be reversed.

The Gerson Therapy has shown that it is able to stop bone loss and regenerate bones already weakened by osteoporosis. The therapy also heals and regenerates all other organ systems.

Osteoporosis Drugs Making Bones Brittle

In his book, *The Health Revolution*, **Ross Horne explains, "Together with inactivity, high protein intake causes osteoporosis, weak and porous bones.** With a daily high protein intake, the body goes into negative mineral balance because of high acidity. In the UK, tests have shown that vegetarians aged 70 have bones equal to or of greater density than the bones of meat eaters aged 50. Calcium compounds and supplements can cause calcification of the aorta and serious damage to circulation."[16] [Emphasis added.]

Ross Horne goes further, stating, "One of the main reasons for that condition [osteoporosis] is that calcium is withdrawn from the bones in an effort by the body to neutralize acids formed as a result of excess dietary [animal] protein."[17] [Emphasis added.]

The process by which this occurs is as follows: When you eat a good-sized portion of animal protein (any animal protein), your body extracts its food value and leaves the rest to be eliminated. This part is called "ash" because, like ash left over after a fire, it is the part that cannot be used as fuel. The ash from animal protein is high in phosphorous, which, when it combines with water in your body, creates phosphoric acid. The result of eating animal protein, then, is the creation of acid in your system, and the gradual lowering of your pH level (the acid-alkaline balance). The lower the pH, the more acid your system is. There are other sources of acidity in the standard diet, but cutting out animal proteins is one of the easiest to accomplish.

Our physiological processes, however, are exquisitely sensitive to variations in the pH from its ideal, slightly alkaline, value of 7.35-7.36. (A pH of 7.0 is "neutral.") Many of our vital functions start to fail when the pH is out of range, as evidenced by loss of consciousness due to hyperventilation, for example. When the pH starts to drop due to the consumption of animal protein, your body systems go into emergency mode to restore us to healthy (alkaline) levels.

In order to return an acidic system to alkalinity, the body must find a source of alkaline material to introduce into the mix. The largest and most readily available source of such material is the calcium carbonate contained in your skeletal structure, the bones. Faced with an existential (life-threatening) situation, your system will "borrow" some calcium from the skeleton, and count on you to replace it in the near future. All too often, our dietary habits dictate another meal high in animal protein, then yet another.

This constant "borrowing" of calcium from our bones without replacing it eventually leads to osteoporosis, since over a lifetime of such abuse, we are capable of removing up to 75% of the necessary structural calcium from our bone mass, often with familiar catastrophic results: hip fractures, collapsed spinal vertebrae, brittle bones and an extremely painful inability of the bones to sustain healthy posture or activity.

The prevention and corrective remedy for this kind of damage is a plant-based diet, rich in the calcium from natural foods, that is accompanied by the enzymes and co-factors necessary for the calcium to be properly metabolized and incorporated into the skeletal structure for the repair task.

REFERENCES

1. "Osteoporosis" (http://generalhealthtopics.com/osteoporosis-509.html).
2. "The Mouth-Body Connection" (www.greaterphoenixpi.com/periodontal-disease/mouth-body-connection.asp).
3. "Osteoporosis" (www.ncbi.nlm.nih.gov/pubmedhealth/PMH0001400/).
4. John Robbins, *Diet for a New America* (Walpole, NH: Stillpoint Publishing, 1987); Ross Horne, *The Heath Revolution* (Avalon Beach, N.S.W. Australia: Happy Landings Pty. Ltd., 1984).
5. Blake More, Spectrum, *Yoga Journal*, Mar.–Apr. 1996, p.18.
6. Ibid.
7. Ibid.
8. Ibid.
9. S. Altschuler, "Dietary Protein and Calcium Loss: A Review," *Nutritional Research* 2:193-200, 1982.
10. John Robbins, *May All Be Fed* (New York: Avon Books, 1993), p. 58. Original quote, cited by John Robbins, is J. McDougall, *McDougall's Medicine* (Piscataway, NJ: New Century Publishing, 1985), p. 75
11. Note 4 (Robbins), supra, pp. 193-194.
12. Pablo Alonso-Coello, Alberto López García-Franco, Gordon Guyatt and Ray Moynihan, "Drugs for pre-osteoporosis: prevention or disease mongering?"*BMJ* 336 : 126 doi: 10.1136/bmj.39435.656250.AD 17 Jan 2008.
13. Dr. Mercola, "Did Merck Hide the Risks of Fosamax?" July 25, 2007 (http://articles.mercola.com/sites/articles/archive/2007/07/25/did-merck-hide-the-risks-of-fosamax.aspx).
14. Brad Case, DC, *Thugs, Drugs and the War on Bugs* (Prunedale, CA: New Renaissance Books, 2010), p. 104.
15. Adriane Fugh-Berman and Charlea T. Massion, "Bone-Breaking Drugs?" *Women's Health Activist Newsletter*, Sep./Oct. 2008.
16. Ross Horne, *The Health Revolution* (Avalon Beach, N.S.W, Australia: Happy Landings Pty Ltd, 1984), p. 145.
17. R. Horne, *The Health Revolution, Third edition* (Sydney, Australia: Harper Collins Publishers, 1984), p. 325.

PART II

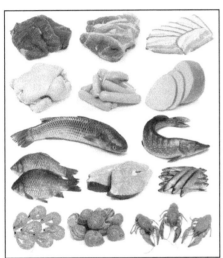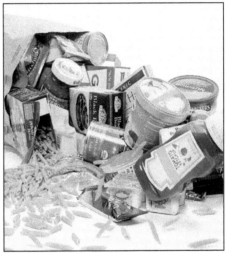

Origins and Causes

CHAPTER 8

The Cure Is in the Cause

T he title of this chapter, taken from a book with the same name by Dr. Ruza Bogdanovich, ND, PhD[1] (www.thecureisinthecause.com) immediately raises the question, "What does it mean?"

The idea is simple and logical—as all great truths must be. It means that, in order to truly heal (or cure) a physical problem, you must first understand the cause. You can then remove or alter the underlying condition, the cause, and resolve the problem.

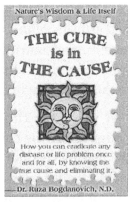

There are many books, medical texts, in-depth research reports, extensive descriptions of pathologies and, especially in arthritis (or other bone diseases), many different types of rheumatic diseases available for study. Nevertheless, in spite of decades and millions of dollars spent on research, *Taber's Cyclopedic Medical Dictionary,*[2] along with the volumes on arthritis, identify numerous possible causes, but no clear or definitive cause.[3] Thus, the often-proposed explanation of genetic predisposition is exposed as a guess rather than a scientific fact. Inflammation is usually present; however, the cause of that inflammation is unknown or not mentioned.

So let us return to our chapter title phrase. If the cause is not known, how can we produce a cure? In many reports, the use of methotrexate is recommended for people suffering from rheumatoid arthritis. Methotrexate (in larger doses) is a chemotherapy drug and diminishes (and/or suppresses) the immune response. It has reportedly alleviated the distress of rheumatoid arthritis for a short time—since it reduces inflammation—but it makes the patient seriously ill. Many patients receiving this drug eventually refuse to continue taking it.

These patients have two simple explanations: It stops working after the first few weeks, and the side effects are severe and include suppression of bone marrow function, hepatitis, stomach pain, debilitation, nausea and hair loss.[4] In view of the above, it is imperative to address and remove the cause. Clearly, since rheumatoid arthritis is not caused by a deficiency of chemotherapy, administering these drugs does not cure the disease!

We are going to examine a subject that is almost never mentioned in the literature and research regarding either osteoarthritis or rheumatoid arthritis: *nutrition.* Many assumptions are made about nutrition by medical and nutritional "experts." One of the principal ones, and the worst offender, is that human beings absolutely require animal proteins for health, strength and well-being.

If we take a close look at the human body, we see that it is not designed for the consumption of animal products. Our teeth are not the tearing teeth of meat-eating animals but are instead the grinding teeth of vegetarians. Our stomach acid is not adequate for the digestion of meat, fish or fowl, nor even of milk and milk products such as cheese. Meat-eating animals have about seven times the amount of stomach acid as the human body produces. Further, our small intestine is very long, like that of other vegetarian animals, for the purpose of extracting the minerals and nutrients contained in a plant-based diet.

Animal products, on the other hand, contain no fiber, so the bowel required for a carnivore is shorter and doesn't move as well. Another problem is that the digestion of meat leaves a toxic residue that remains too long in the human intestinal tract, and tends to allow these poisons to be reabsorbed into the bloodstream. They further damage the friendly bacteria that should be produced in a healthy colon. Thus the consumption of meat and other animal products is largely responsible for colon cancer as well as other chronic diseases.[5]

The well-known nutritionist and author, John H. Tobe, writes, "For approximately fifty years we have been told that milk is the perfect food. Believe me, a myth it is. It has no basis in scientific data, fact, experience, or test. In fact there is loads of evidence available to prove that it is not a good food, a healthful food, or even a suitable food for human beings."[6]

How do other vertebrate animals behave? Like us, they give birth to live young, who depend on their mother's milk for their first nutrition. However, when the offspring is weaned, it is never again fed milk—certainly not the milk of other species.[7]

Eastern countries use more agricultural products for feeding their populations. They live mainly on fruit, vegetables and grains.[8] Dr. Ruza states, "**According to the *Code of Manu*, the world's oldest human law compiled several thousand years ago in India and still the principal law of Hinduism, the use of cow's milk is prohibited.** The Japanese rarely used the milk of any animals. Their use of cow's milk was introduced to Japan from China in about 800 AD and continued for a short time. However the use of milk soon faded because the environment of Japan was not suited for raising cows, and *because ill health developed quickly among milk users.*"[9] [Emphasis added.]

For years, Danny Vierra[10] has successfully used a nutritional healing method with many people and gathered valuable experiences. In a Dec. 31, 2010 e-mail, he writes: "**The late Dr. Virgil Hulse, DDS, once told me that as a Milk and Dairy inspector for 13 years in California, he found 80% of the herds had cows with leukemia and 50% of the herds had cows with Bovine AIDS.** This was in the county in which I live. Milk Does A Body Good? Instead, drink water or fresh juices when thirsty. The FDA allows 750 million pus cells per liter of milk to be transported in interstate commerce."[11] [Emphasis added.]

Let's examine one case of rheumatoid arthritis to try and discern a possible "cause" for its onset. Deanna was a high school athlete in her late teens. Her trainer suggested that she drink a lot of milk to strengthen her muscles and give her a good supply of calcium. Within a year, in 1970, she started to suffer from rheumatoid arthritis.

Deanna's joints became progressively more inflamed and swollen, then developed lumps and calcifications. In spite of treatments with gold and prednisone, she was bedfast by 1976. She was in constant pain and had stiffness in all her joints: fingers, knuckles, wrists, elbows, knees and ankles, with bony deformities. She had great difficulty walking, in addition to suffering from heart palpitations and labored breathing. She was pale, anemic and hypoglycemic. Fifteen to 20 aspirins a day only took the sharp edge off her pain, which was constant, and prevented her from sleeping. She stated, "I feel like a prisoner in my own body."

Deanna started the Gerson Therapy at the Mexican hospital in May 1979. In six weeks, she was virtually free of pain, most of her lumps were dissolving and her frozen wrists started to move. Eventually, all her problems were resolved, except that a few joints were not quite clear. By 1981, she was water skiing. Fourteen years later, she had excellent energy, was active, got married and started a family.

While adding milk products to the diet can seriously contribute to the cause of RA, unfortunately simply removing it is not sufficient to cure this terrible disease.

Would You Believe: Milk—the White Poison?

The following is a report on the study entitled "White Poison: The Horrors of Milk," published by Shanti Rangwani, MD, a columnist for the *Times of India*.[12] I take no credit for any of the following material; it is strictly work written and published by Dr. Rangwani.

In the *Gerson Healing Newsletter*,[13] we have published the work of Professor T. Colin Campbell, whose research clearly demonstrates that milk, along with all animal proteins, is seriously harmful to our health. **Where there is little or no milk and where people live on vegetarian foods or a vegan diet, there is virtually no chronic disease, especially no cancer!**

However, Dr. Rangwani goes a great deal further, not only in his research, but in his conclusions about the dangers of milk. **He reports that drinking milk, according to medical research, is likely to cause anemia, migraine, bloating, gas, indigestion, asthma, prostate cancer and a host of potentially fatal allergies.**[14]

Why do U.S. consumers not hear these facts? The U.S. government ignored this research and declares milk "essential to good health."[15] It even subsidizes the milk industry to the tune of billions of dollars and requires milk in its public school programs.[16] Celebrities, in advertising campaigns, tell us that milk is rich in proteins, calcium and vitamins. Milk used to be decried only by naturopaths and vegans; however, now the damage to our health by milk is being stressed by many mainstream doctors.

Dr. Rangwani continues by reporting that the former chairman of pediatrics at Johns Hopkins University, Frank Oski, MD, published a book titled *Don't Drink Your Milk.*[17] In the book, Oski blames every second health problem kids develop on hormone-ridden commercial milk, as well as 60% of ear infections in children under six years of age. It is apparently even the #1 cause of iron-deficiency anemia in infants, according to the American Association of Pediatrics.[18]

Milk is particularly poorly handled by African Americans and most Latinos, Asians and southern Europeans. They are apparently deficient in lactase (the enzyme needed to digest milk). In other words, most of the world's population is not biologically equipped to digest milk! Dr. Rangwani states, "Milk does no body good, but for the vast majority of the world's people—people of color—it is a public health disaster."[19]

"No other animal drinks cow's milk, not even calves once they are weaned."[20] **Dr. Benjamin Spock, the leading authority on child care in the United States, warned against "feeding cow's glue to children"[21] since it can pave the way for so many serious diseases in the future.** [Emphasis added.]

The U.S. Department of Agriculture (USDA) continues to require that school lunch programs include milk, always stressing that it contains calcium[22]—in spite of the hundreds of studies that show an increase in osteoporosis and bone breakage in people who consume milk.[23] (The calcium contained in milk is not absorbed by the body.) The powerful dairy lobby also perpetuates the lies to continue to receive government price support for this "health food."[24] The government pays over a billion dollars a year for surplus butter.[25]

"Dr. Robert Cohen of the Dairy Education Board, a nonprofit organization dedicated to exposing the milk lobby, contends that the dramatic 52% rise in asthma deaths among minority kids in New York coincides with the surplus milk, cheese and butter pumped into them under the USDA free school lunch programs," states Dr. Rangwani.[26]

The controversial recombinant bovine growth hormone (rBGH) is banned in many countries.[27] In 1959, the highest average annual milk production per cow was 7,192 lb. per cow and, in 2010, the highest average annual milk production was approximately 22,000 lb. per cow, an increase of about 206%.[28] The milk is likely to contain pus from the cows' udders since the hormone promotes mastitis. Dairy farmers treat this BGH-caused infection with heavy doses of antibiotics. This increases the germ's tolerance and decreases the effectiveness of antibiotics in humans.

Estimates show that 38% of milk in the United States is "contaminated with sulfa drugs or other antibiotics," according to a study by the Centre for Science in the Public Interest and published in the Wall Street Journal.[29] [Emphasis added.]

Dr. Rangwani states, "There is also a direct link between milk consumption and prostate cancer among African Americans, who have the highest incidence of this disease in the world.[30] A study published in *Cancer* (a journal of the American Cancer Society) has shown that men who reported drinking three or more glasses of whole milk daily had a higher risk for prostate cancer than men who reported never drinking whole milk.[31]

Dr. Rangwani concludes his report by stating that the dairy lobby continues to get the ear of most medical practitioners to promote their "drink milk" propaganda.[32] All of the 1,500 studies listed in *Medicine*[33] deal with the pus, blood, antibiotics and carcinogens in milk while not one points to its "goodness."

Mothers, totally convinced of the "goodness" of milk, and imbued with the propaganda that their kids need milk, are at a loss on how to replace milk in their children's diet. Meanwhile, new propaganda has opened the door to soy milk! Soy products have been heavily promoted by industry and the stories being publicized are also full of half-truths and lies.

Soy products contain phytic acid, a substance that blocks the absorption of other nutrients from the gut, thus making other foods useless and promoting nutrient deficiencies![34] Soy products do *not* prevent cancer.

So, what to do? We suggest the best possible alternative: namely, juice made from organic carrots, apples and citrus fruits. Avoid dry cereals for children and give them freshly cooked oatmeal with a fruit sauce—similar to custard with a delicious topping. Completely avoid cow's milk as well as soy milk for your children's sake.

REFERENCES

1. Dr. Ruza Bogdanovich, ND, PhD, *The Cure is in the Cause: Nature's Wisdom and Life Itself* (Genoa, NV: Spirit Spring Foundation, Inc., 2001), pp. 60-61. The chapter title is taken with permission from her book. Her website is www.thecureisinthecause.com.
2. *Taber's Cyclopedic Medical Dictionary, 20th edition* (Philadelphia: F. A. Davis Company, 2005).
3. Note 2 (*Taber's*), supra, p. 173.
4. "Methotrexate Side Effects" (www.drugs.com/sfx/methotrexate-side-effects.html).
5. J. Kreuning, *Colorectal Cancer* (The Hague, Netherlands: Martinus Nijhoff Publishers bv., 1980), p. 86.
6. Robert Cohen, *Milk—The Deadly Poison* (Oradell, NJ: Argus Publishing, 1997); Note 1 (Bogdanovich), supra, pp. 60-61.
7. Note 1 (Bogdanovich), supra, pp. 60-61.
8. Ibid., p. 59.
9. Ibid.

10. Danny Vierra is the Director of Modern Manna Ministries (www.modernmanna.com) and BellaVita Lifestyle Center. He is a dynamic, international speaker who specializes in detoxification programs, alternative therapies and natural medicine. He is also the founder of Modern Manna Health Crusade (annual convention), a pastor, a health food store owner and a healer.

11. Personal correspondence to the author, Dec. 31, 2010. "To ensure high-quality dairy products, BTSCCs are monitored in milk shipments using standards outlined in the U.S. Pasteurized Milk Ordinance. The legal maximum BTSCC for 'Grade A' milk shipments is 750,000 cells/mL." This translates to 750 million pus cells per liter (www.aphis.usda.gov/animal_health/nahms/dairy/downloads/dairy_monitoring/BTSCC_2008infosheet.pdf).

12. Shanti Rangwani, MD, columnist for the *Times of India,* from "White Poison: The Horrors of Milk" (Dec. 3, 2001). More details can be found at www.alternet.org/story/12002.

13. Professor T. Colin Campbell, "A Report on Nutrition Studies, *Gerson Healing Newsletter,* Vol. 17-3, May/June 2002.

14. Note 12 (Rangwani), supra.

15. "The government declares that milk is essential to good health, and subsidizes the milk industry to the tune of billions of dollars, and requires milk in its public school lunch programs." (www.healthandnutritionbasics.com/arogosienski/article-detail.php?Health-and-Nutrition-Basics-Article-Milk-The-Dangerous-Truth-About-Dairy-Products-41).

16. "Dairy Program Subsidies in the United States totaled $4.8 billion from 1995-2009." (http://farm.ewg.org/progdetail.php?fips=00000&progcode=dairy); Physicians Committee for Responsible Medicine, "The Need for Alternatives to Cow's Milk in the National School Lunch Program": "The National School Lunch Act requires that schools participating in the National School Lunch Program always offer cow's milk in order to receive federal reimbursement." (www.healthyschoollunches.org/changes/non-dairy.cfm).

17. Frank A. Oski, MD, *Don't Drink Your Milk!: New Frightening Medical Facts About the World's Most Overrated Nutrient* (Ringgold, GA: Teach Services, 1992).

18. Note 12 (Rangwani), supra. "Milk consumption is the number one cause of iron-deficiency in infants today according to the American Association of Pediatrics" (www.healthandnutritionbasics.com/arogosienski/article-

detail.php?Health-and-Nutrition-Basics-Article-Milk-The-Dangerous-Truth-About-Dairy-Products-41); A. Carley, "Anemia: When Is it Iron Deficiency?" *Prevention,* "A diet including cow's milk in the first year of life has been suggested as the major risk factor for subsequent development of iron deficiency and anemia in childhood (Kazal, 2002), therefore elimination of this risk factor is an important component of preventive care."; "Whole milk should not be used before 12 completed months of age." (http://aappolicy.aappublications.org/cgi/content/full/pediatrics;126/5/1040) from the American Association of Pediatrics.

19. Note 12 (Rangwani), supra.
20. "The Dangerous Truth About Dairy Products" (www.healthandnutritionbasics.com/arogosienski/article-detail.php?Health-and-Nutrition-Basics-Article-Milk-The-Dangerous-Truth-About-Dairy-Products-41).
21. Note 12 (Rangwani), supra. "The late Dr. Benjamin Spock, the U.S.'s leading authority on child care, spoke out against feeding 'cow's glue' to children, saying it can cause anemia, allergies, and diabetes and in the long term, will set kids up for obesity and heart disease, the number one cause of death in this country." (www.purewatergazette.net/whitepoison.htm); www.healthandnutritionbasics.com/arogosienski/article-detail.php?Health-and-Nutrition-Basics-Article-Milk-The-Dangerous-Truth-About-Dairy-Products-41).
22. Note 12 (Rangwani), supra.
23. John Robbins, *Diet for a New America* (Walpole, NH: Stillpoint Publishing, 1987), p. 199. Robbins says that these studies show that milk "appears actually to **contribute** to the accelerating development of osteoporosis." [Emphasis from the author.]
24. Note 12 (Rangwani), supra.
25. Ibid. "The dairy lobby perpetrates lies to ensure its profits. It benefits directly from the exaggerated support prices the government shells out for this 'health food.' The government pays over a billion dollars a year for surplus butter." (www.purewatergazette.net/whitepoison.htm).
26. Note 12 (Rangwani), supra.
27. "Since 1994, every industrialized country in the world, except for the US, has banned the drug." (www.shirleys-wellness-cafe.com/bgh.htm).
28. U.S. Department of Agriculture, "Milk Production" (1959–1963) (http://usda.mannlib.cornell.edu/usda/nass/MilkProd/1960s/1965/MilkProd-10-12-1965.pdf; "Overview of the United States Dairy Industry"

(2009) (http://usda.mannlib.cornell.edu/usda/current/USDairyIndus/USDairyIndus-09-22-2010.pdf).

29. Centre for Science in the Public Interest and published in the *Wall Street Journal,* Dec. 29, 1989.
30. Note 12 (Rangwani), supra.
31. C. Mettlin, S. Selenskas, N. Natarajan and R. Huben, "Beta-carotene and animal fats and their relationship to prostate cancer risk. A case-control study," *Cancer* 1989 Aug 1;64(3):605-12.
32. Note 12 (Rangwani), supra.
33. Shanti Rangwani, "White Poison," Dec. 15, 2001 (http://colorlines.com/archives/2001/12/white_poison.html).
34. C. Gerson and B. Bishop, *Healing the Gerson Way: Defeating Cancer and Other Chronic Diseases* (Carmel, CA: Totality Books, 2007), p. 148.

CHAPTER 9

Breakdown of the Body's Defenses

It is interesting to note that, when people are told they need "protein," only foods of animal origin come to mind, including meat, fish, poultry, eggs and processed dairy products. All animal protein on the planet originally derives from plant protein, and the belief that we need "complete protein" is a long-discarded myth, perpetuated by the meat industry for its own marketing purposes. If one follows their flawed logic to its conclusion, the best protein—the most "complete" for human consumption—would be other humans! In addition, animal protein that we consume is almost always heat-damaged, since it is consumed cooked, baked or, worst of all, deep fried. Milk is pasteurized and not sold in raw form. For these reasons, animal proteins are poorly assimilated and mostly harmful to the human organism.[1]

Food originates in the soil. Dr. Gerson called the soil "our external metabolism."[2] We must live on the products of the earth but we persist in poisoning this, our main source of food and health! In the past 130 years, artificial fertilizers have superseded the natural replacement of minerals after crops draw nutrients from the soil. These fertilizers are unnatural products of synthesis and, above all, only partly nourish the soil. They consist essentially of three elements: nitrogen, phosphorus and potassium (NPK). That could be a good start, **but we have to understand that plants (and our bodies) require some 52 different minerals. Where, for example, are the iron, calcium, magnesium, manganese, iodine and all the others? Missing! The resulting plants are severely deficient, growing in soil lacking trace minerals essential to their well-being.**

Because of their mineral deficiency, plants are unable to produce their normal defenses. Fungi, bugs and viruses attack the crops, so farmers demand help from the chemical companies, who happily supply fungicides, pesticides and growth stimulants that guarantee enormous present and future profits for the manufacturers, not the farmers.

The result is that our commercial produce retains toxic residues from pesticides and fungicides, and is increasingly genetically modified. Farmers come under severe financial stress because of their rising dependence on expensive petroleum-based chemicals and the ever-increasing forced use of **"terminator seeds."** These are specially designed to grow for only one season, forcing farmers to purchase new seeds for each new planting.

When Dr. Gerson realized that animal proteins were harmful and, when consumed in excess, at least partly responsible for the onset of chronic disease,[3] he introduced organic, plant-based general nutrition, freshly prepared and salt free, to initiate healing.

Not only is our modern plant-based food toxic and of poor quality because it is grown in poisoned and deficient soil, it is also processed, flavored, canned, jarred, bottled, preserved, frozen, colored and boxed—for "convenience."

In the course of processing, large numbers of chemical additives are introduced, all certified by the Food and Drug Administration (FDA) as "GRAS" (generally recognized as safe) when, in fact, they have never been adequately tested and proven to be safe! **Among these are fluoride, genetically modified organisms, mercury-bearing additives to food and vaccines, MSG (monosodium glutamate), Aspartame (NutraSweet) and many others. The more than 3,000 total sub-**

stances together comprise an inventory often referred to as "Everything" Added to Food in the United States (EAFUS).[4]

One seriously damaging additive is salt (sodium chloride). People are so used to adding salt to their food that they find it difficult to eat anything unsalted! This is understandable since almost all the food is grown in deficient soil and then boiled in lots of water. When the water is thrown out, the flavor goes with it, as well as any remaining food value. In spite of repeated warnings about the danger of using salt, its consumption is extremely high—even higher in the United States than in European countries.[5]

Salt forces the body to retain water, which it uses to dilute the toxic effect of sodium in the cells. This results in edema of the tissues. Salt damages the kidneys and the digestive process, so the body is unable to readily absorb calcium.[6]

Most people are not aware that such disturbances cause the body to be unable to use foods, which then act as toxins (poisons). Toxins are also defined as "enzyme inhibitors," further interfering with normal metabolism. Is it surprising that some of the complex body systems fail?

Here is an important consideration: As we have specifically noted in a number of patients, arthritic problems are often associated with kidney dysfunction. It is important to understand that, among other activities, kidneys are involved in excreting the end products of protein digestion and sodium; in other words, they are very important detoxifying organs. Therefore, with poor kidney function, these end products are not adequately excreted and cause a great deal of toxicity, pain and "inflammation."[7]

Toxicity and Nutritional Deficiency

Toxicity

Toxicity starts in the soil and in the plants that grow in it. Highly poisonous pesticides, fungicides, herbicides and other chemicals used in commercial agriculture, often until the day of harvesting, leave residues on the plants that become our food. Many of these poisons are systemic (i.e., they permeate the produce and cannot be removed by washing). Unless we eat only organically grown foods, our daily intake is richly laced with a cocktail of agrochemicals whose cumulative effect has never been tested.[8] Additional toxins are introduced by a huge variety of food additives, none of which is safe.

While the public knows that salt is "not good for you," they rarely think of restricting it. The average American diet is unusually high in salt (sodium). This excess interferes with normal body functions and is more than "not good for you"—it is actually toxic.[9]

Professor T. Colin Campbell showed that excess animal protein damages our internal organs and promotes both malignant and non-malignant chronic diseases much more powerfully than the most potent carcinogenic toxins.[10] Our natural nutrition should be vegetarian but it has evolved into a very high animal protein diet. Animals are inadequately raised, with artificial foods, chemical growth promoters, hormones and antibiotics. As we age, we are less able to digest the high level of animal proteins in our diet while the poorly digested products become toxins and interfere with normal functions. The animal fats that are part of almost all meat, poultry and milk products similarly are less well digested as the body ages and enzymes are no longer as effective.

In addition to those in our food, there are poisons in the air from many sources: car exhausts and industry, including tiny particles released by tires. Toxic substances are added to the water, including chlorine and fluoride.

The body attempts to rid itself of all these substances to protect its integrity. However, it is now faced with the additional problem of deficiency, which severely limits its capacity to deal with this load of toxins.

Nutritional Deficiency

Deficient food grows in poor quality soil. For well over 150 years, artificial fertilizers have been increasingly used in commercial agriculture, providing the soil with three major elements: nitrogen, phosphorus and potassium (NPK). They do not provide the more than 50 minerals and trace elements essential in keeping the soil healthy, fertile and rich in enzymes and microorganisms, which characterize naturally fertilized, humus-rich land. The resulting impoverished soil can only produce deficient, nutrient-poor plants, which become our equally deficient daily food.[11]

A number of the rheumatoid pathologies fall into the category of collagen diseases. "Collagen" is a strong, fibrous, insoluble protein contained in connective tissue, including skin, tendons, ligaments, bone and cartilage.[12] Standard medical dogma blames rheumatic diseases on an "overactive immune system." As a result, they are classified as "autoimmune diseases," and include:

- rheumatoid arthritis
- lupus erythematosus
- scleroderma
- mixed collagen disease

We feel strongly that "autoimmune" disease does not exist. In diseases described as such, allopathic medicine claims that the body's immune system turns against itself and destroys it own tissue! Successful application of the Gerson Therapy has proved over and over— in *all* the above diseases—that this is a faulty observation.

On the contrary, the Gerson Therapy, which clearly activates and *increases* the body's immune responses, demonstrates that these diseases are quite readily *curable* by immune enhancement. It becomes obvious that the body is not attacking its own *healthy* tissue but is only breaking down and eliminating sick and damaged cells or organ systems. Therefore, an increased activity of the immune system is the result—*not the cause*—of chronic, so-called "autoimmune" diseases!

The conclusions drawn from the above are that, in orthodox medicine, the causes of degenerative diseases are either unknown or they are misunderstood and mislabeled (and therefore incorrectly treated). Thus, the diseases are considered "incurable" and only symptoms are treated and essentially suppressed.

Earlier we mentioned a few of the aggressively toxic and damaging factors that lead to disease. **If toxicity and deficiency are, as Dr. Gerson maintained, the two major causes of degenerative problems, they are necessarily the two main areas needing to be addressed for healing. If the body is sick due to toxicity and deficiency, in order to heal, one must** *detoxify* **as well as** *intensively restore nutrients.*

While food is deficient, it is further depleted by processing. All canned, jarred, boxed, preserved, bottled and otherwise prepared items are damaged by high heat and preservatives, and contain little nutrition. **If our food were truly nutritious, our bodies would be better able to deal with toxicity, but it is not. As a result, the degenerative process sets in, opening the door to serious chronic disease.**

Processed foods are also depleted of vitamins and enzymes.[13] Enzymes are destroyed at a temperature of 140° F[14] and can only be supplied to the body via raw food such as fruit and raw salads and their fresh juices. Few people consume enough of these to supply adequate quantities of enzymes and vitamins for a healthy system.

It is clear that the above problems have to be dealt with in order to initiate healing.

Significant Contributing Factors

Chemical Agriculture

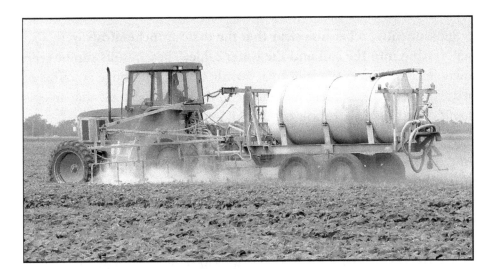

Artificial fertilizers have been in increasing use for well over 150 years, damaging and impoverishing the soil and the microorganisms on which the health of the soil and of all plant life depends. Plants, in turn, are the food of animals and humans, and their reduced nutritional value has far-reaching effects. Dr. Gerson was one of the few visionary scientists who realized early on that there was a definite link between dietary deficiencies and diseases—and between diseases and a sick, depleted soil. He wrote, **"There is an external and an internal metabolism upon which all life depends; both are closely and inextricably connected with each other; furthermore, the reserves of both are not inexhaustible."**[15]

Once the reserves of the soil are exhausted, the plants begin to sicken. Deficient in nutrients, they lose their defenses against pests, rust, fungi and a multitude of other invaders. Hence, fungicides, pesticides and other toxic chemicals have been developed. At the beginning it was assumed that these agrochemicals were harmless if applied "as directed"; unfortunately, this has not proved to be the case.

The heavy pesticides—specifically DDT (dichloro-diphenyl-trichlo-roethane)—were first distributed halfway through World War II, around 1943. As Dr. Gerson reports in his book,[16] this and other toxic materials were found in meat, butter, milk and even mother's milk within 18 months!

Subsequently, it became clear that the toxic agrochemicals were also penetrating into the soil and the water table. These results can be seen today in several areas of California, heavily treated with huge amounts of pesticides every year, where the water and the soil are so toxic that an epidemic of primary liver cancer has hit children who played outdoors.[17]

The situation has gone from bad to worse. After DDT had been used for some time, the insect pests became resistant to it, so that heavier, even more toxic materials, such as dieldrin, had to be produced. At the same time, it transpired that the human body was *not* able to develop a resistance to those poisons. **Their effect on adults is bad enough; tragically, embryos, tiny babies and small children with their delicate constitutions suffer more serious damage to their developing bodies.**

Though there is no "proof" that glyphosates, the most widely used weed killer in the world, have caused cancer, *Lancet Oncology* reports that a number of recent studies have shown a strong probability that glyphosate (the "active" ingredient of RoundUp) is carcinogenic and have thus classified it as a Class 2A carcinogen, "probably carcinogenic to humans."[18] Monsanto vigorously denies the allegation, calling it "outrageous," with no data to back it up.[19]

Quite the opposite, in fact. Independent studies in 1980 and 1981 showed that there was a connection between glyphosates and cancer formation, but Monsanto, in collusion with the Environmental Protection Agency (EPA), suppressed release of this information, calling it "trade secrets."[20] Thus, Monsanto has known about the deleterious effects of RoundUp on human health for over 35 years and has hidden that information.

In March 2015, 17 experts from 11 countries met at the International Agency for Research on Cancer (IARC) in Lyon, France, to assess the carcinogenicity of the organophosphate pesticides tetrachlorvinphos, parathion, malathion, diazinon, and glyphosate (table). These assessments will be published as volume 112 of the IARC Monographs.[21]

More and more independent studies of RoundUp are showing that, contrary to Monsanto's claims of RoundUp safety, it is actually 125 times as toxic as previously believed.[22] Additionally, the "inert" ingredients in RoundUp actually serve to significantly enhance the toxicity of glyphosate.[23] Independent studies not funded by Monsanto and 50 other governments have declared glyphosate toxic to human cells.[24]

MIT researcher Stephanie Seneff, PhD, has spent 30 years publishing articles on biology and technology. At a recent conference, she noted that the side effects of autism closely mimic those of glyphosate toxicity, and showed a strong correlation between the use of RoundUp on crops, the rise of GMO RoundUp-ready crops and the rapid rise in autism. "At today's rate, by 2025, one in two children will be autistic."[25]

Monsanto depends on studies by scientists they have funded to show the safety of their deadly products.

As if dealing with the existing problems caused by agrochemicals were not enough, human health is facing the further threat posed by genetically modified organism (GMO) food. This is an area where the conflict between powerful commercial interests and public health has come out into the open, despite GMO-producer Monsanto's best efforts to suppress data casting serious doubts on the safety of GMO foods for human consumption.[26] This is in keeping with the normal routine of agrochemical manufacturers who invariably set out to prove, by hook or by crook, the "safety" of one or another of their products. **Anyone on an average modern diet is bound to consume the residues of several toxic substances clinging to fruits and vegetables, yet no one has ever researched the cumulative effect of this kind of toxic cocktail.**

The picture is gloomy, yet all is not lost. From small beginnings, the organic production of fruits and vegetables has grown exponentially in recent years, allowing the enlightened consumer to live on poison-free produce. **Organic food, grown on traditionally fertilized soil, has the further advantage of containing all the minerals, trace elements,**

enzymes and vitamins needed for good health. This is why, in order to achieve healing, Gerson patients must use nothing but organic produce.

Enough has been said to illustrate the vicious circle initiated by the average modern diet. When living on toxin-rich but nutrient-poor food—especially "fast food"—people begin to suffer from headaches, arthritis, insomnia, depression, frequent colds, infections, digestive problems and more. They use more over-the-counter drugs, while doctors prescribe symptom-relieving medicines, which don't deal with the underlying cause of their disease.

Drugs

When the metabolism is seriously disturbed, symptoms appear, most frequently pain. Of course, in rheumatism or osteoarthritis, there is swelling, lumps, interference with normal joint function, stiffness and often weakness. At that point, the affected person goes to a physician to get help, hoping for a cure. The patient will be given a mild painkiller until such time as the disease worsens and the pain becomes more severe. In most cases, the patient will not be told that the doctor has no cure and can only relieve symptoms.

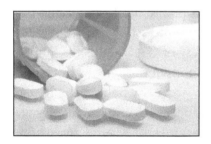

Generally, however, the problem doesn't start locally. **The patient has damaged his or her body with animal proteins, fats, salt, fast foods, possibly smoking, alcohol and drugs such as antibiotics to fight infections, sleeping pills and antidepressants. All these create toxicity in the body, damaging systems and functions and causing arthritis or other chronic[27] disease processes to begin.**

Aside from the two major types of arthritis—rheumatoid arthritis and osteoarthritis—there are a number of others. Each type is treated with different drugs, a lengthy list of pain relievers. The problem is that virtually all of these pain-relief drugs, certainly the most popular, are highly toxic and have severe side effects, including heart attack and death, as evidenced by the long lists of effects noted by their manufacturers.[28]

Some of the drugs—the so-called nonsteroidal anti-inflammatory drugs (NSAIDs)—are routinely used because, in most cases of arthritis, inflammation is present. "Conservative calculations estimate that approximately 107,000 patients hospitalized annually for nonsteroidal anti-inflammatory drug (NSAID)-related gastrointestinal (GI) complications and at least 16,500 NSAID-related deaths occur each year among arthritis patients alone. The figures of all NSAID users would be overwhelming, yet the scope of this problem is generally under-appreciated."[29]

In June 1999, in the prestigious *New England Journal of Medicine,* there is a similar statement: **"It has been estimated conservatively that 16,500 NSAID-related deaths occur among patients with rheumatoid arthritis or osteoarthritis every year in the United States.** This figure is similar to the number of deaths from the acquired immunodeficiency syndrome and considerably greater than the number of deaths from multiple myeloma, asthma, cervical cancer, or Hodgkin's disease. If deaths from gastrointestinal toxic effects from NSAIDs were tabulated separately in the National Vital Statistics reports, these effects would constitute the 15th most common cause of death in the United States. Yet these toxic effects remain mainly a 'silent epidemic,' with many physicians and most patients unaware of the magnitude of the problem. Furthermore the mortality statistics do not include deaths ascribed to the use of over-the-counter NSAIDS."[30] [Emphasis added.]

One such drug—VIOXX, marketed by Merck—was in the news in 2004. Unlike NSAIDS, it doesn't cause stomach ulcers, internal bleeding and death; instead, it causes heart attacks and strokes.[31] **VIOXX is supposed to be a simple medication for arthritis pain (medically called a "COX-2 selective inhibitor") but, "during the 10 years and four months it was on the market, this one drug caused an estimated 160,000 cases of heart attack and stroke in the U.S. alone and 55,000 deaths."**[32] [Emphasis added.]

NSAIDs pose other problems: "The side effects can include stomach upset and bleeding, kidney and liver damage and water and sodium retention. They also block the body's ability to produce cartilage, and increase the destruction of cartilage lining the ends of the bone. So, in the long term, NSAIDs actually worsen the condition they are pre-scribed to treat."[33]

Other COX-2 inhibitor medications (e.g., Celebrex, marketed by Pfizer) were not removed from the market as VIOXX was. In spite of scientific data, criticisms and ongoing deaths, the FDA allowed VIOXX back on the market![34]

We have only discussed the most harmful drugs and those that have been most publicized. There are many more doctor-prescribed or over-the-counter (OTC) pain-relieving drugs on the market. They are approved by the FDA since the pharmaceutical corporations use their power and deep pockets to "persuade" the researchers to allow them. FDA agents are often recruited from the drug manufacturers and, after serving some time at the FDA, return to their original employers. They are therefore interested in keeping those corporations happy.

The above policies demonstrate that the FDA does not protect the public but only Big Pharma's financial interests. **The *San Francisco Chronicle* quoted the former commissioner of the FDA, Herbert Ley, MD, as follows: "The thing that bugs me is that people think the FDA is protecting them. It isn't. What the FDA is doing and what the public thinks it's doing are as different as night and day."[35]** [Emphasis added.]

What's worse, you can't trust your doctor or his or her drugs to help you eliminate the problems you experience with arthritis and/or other bone diseases because, regarding these pathologies, he or she has been taught that the cause is not known.

Remember: The "cure is in the cause."

Dr. Gerson, on the other hand, reached the conclusion more than 75 years ago that bone, heart and all other chronic diseases have two fundamental causes: toxicity and nutritional deficiency[36] (see "Toxic-ity and Nutritional Deficiency," p. 55). Once he understood this, he was able to devise a cure. With great pleasure, we can say that, in the vast majority of cases, the cure is successful.

The remainder of this book is devoted to describing how it is achieved and how the metabolism can be restored and the body's "healing mechanism" (as Dr. Gerson called it) revived.

We must also remember that pharmaceuticals and inappropriate nutrition are not the only causes of disease. Your body has to deal with the toxic environment, the electromagnetic fields to which we are constantly exposed, the fluoride in our water and polluted air. Stress is also a factor, especially those things that many people do under severely stressful situations: smoke more, take sleeping pills, drink more alcohol and eat fast foods.

Heredity also plays a part, although it has recently been discovered not to be inevitable. "Epigenetics" (the study of changes in the genes) (see Chapter 10, "Epigenetics: The 'New' Science," p. 95) has demonstrated that a proper and healthful diet can correct hereditary problems at the level of the genes.[37]

This is where the Gerson Therapy comes in.

Food Additives

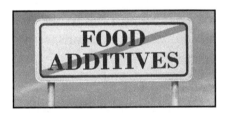

One way of healthy eating goes under the name of the "Stone Age Diet," which says: "Eat only food from which nothing has been removed, to which nothing has been added, and which would go bad if you didn't eat it immediately."[38] You would have a hard time if you tried to find such foods in any supermarket on Earth. What those temples of the food industry sell—unless they have a range of organic produce—is the exact opposite of the above rule.

The ubiquitous use of food additives, whose number is at present about 10,000,[39] serves the sole purpose of making industrially produced foods look better, taste good despite the fact that they contain inferior raw materials, have a longer shelf life and thus be more profitable. Food chemistry is so highly developed that it can mimic almost any natural flavor or scent. What it cannot do is fool the human organism into responding to these fakes as if they were the genuine article, and it only delivers chemicals of varying toxicity instead of essential nutrients.

The most widely used additives include sodium nitrite, saccharin, caffeine, olestra (a fat substitute), artificial colorings and flavorings, antioxidants, emulsifiers, flavor enhancers, thickening agents, aspartame, transfats and MSG—plus unhealthy amounts of sugar, salt and fat. They can cause a multitude of allergic reactions, such as fatigue, behavioral problems, mood swings and, after long-term use, may even lead to heart disease and cancer.

Aspartame

Aspartame deserves special scrutiny, partly because it is in approximately 6,000 food products[40] and is hard to avoid. It is now known to cause a range of serious health problems.

Among long-term regular consumers of aspartame (e.g., in Diet Coke or as NutraSweet in tea and coffee), it can mimic conditions such as multiple sclerosis, diabetes and its complications, arthritis, Alzheimer's disease and severe depression.[41]

These pseudo-diseases are impossible to diagnose and treat, but patients experience immediate relief if they exclude all aspartame-containing foods and drinks from their diet.[42] Since the substance is highly addictive, quitting isn't easy.

Aspartame contains methanol, a cumulative poison, which converts into formaldehyde, a known carcinogen[43]; DKP (diketopiperazine), which in animal experiments has produced brain tumors[44]; and phenylalanine, which can produce severe neurological problems.[45] It is not hard to imagine how it damages the body's defenses.

IMPORTANT NOTE ABOUT EXCESS WEIGHT AND ASPARTAME

Sugar consumption in the United States has been extraordinarily high.[46] People are aware that sugar is a serious cause of weight gain. Chemical manufacturers have learned how to make huge sums of money from this problem by producing artificial sweeteners that add no calories.

One such item is aspartame, known to the public as one of three items: NutraSweet, Equal and Spoonful. When it was first submitted to the U.S. Food and Drug Administration (FDA), their chemists found it so seriously toxic that they would not allow it to be used in foods.[47]

After many more tests[48] plus immense political pressure and maneuvering by Donald Rumsfeld, CEO of aspartame manufacturer Searle, it was finally accepted as safe by the FDA.[49] The additive was approved by the FDA as a result of powerful political pressure, *not safety or product testing!*[50]

Aspartame is seriously neurotoxic and has caused a severe epidemic of a condition that mimics multiple sclerosis, but in an estimated four out of five cases (80%), is simply misdiagnosed aspartame poisoning.[51] Also, if exposed to temperatures above 86° F, it breaks down into methanol (wood alcohol), which is especially toxic for diabetics.[52] It can cause blindness, vertigo, stupor, abdominal pain, convulsions and kidney damage.[53]

Completely aside from these problems, aspartame is a drug that has a "contrary effect." People use "diet drinks" with the hope of consuming sweet drinks without gaining weight. The opposite is true. The Congressional Record has a notation that states, "It makes you crave carbohydrates and will make you FAT."[54]

H. J. Roberts, MD, of the Palm Beach Institute for Medical Research, diabetes specialist and world expert on aspartame, has written against the use of aspartame in his book, *Defense Against Alzheimer's Disease.* He observes that, when he got patients off aspartame, they lost an average of 19.5 pounds.[55] In his book, he also notes that aspartame poisoning is escalating Alzheimer's disease. A hospice nurse observed that some women are now being admitted with Alzheimer's at the age of 30![56]

Dr. Louis Elias, pediatrics professor (Genetics, at Emory University) testified before Congress that, in his original lab tests, animals developed brain tumors from aspartame.[57] When Dr. [Joseph L.] Esposito was lecturing on aspartame, one physician in the audience, a neurosurgeon, said, **"When they remove brain tumors, they have found high levels of aspartame in them."**[58]

There is an excellent replacement product on the market called stevia—a sweet food, not an additive—that actually helps the sugar metabolism and is ideal for diabetics.[59] It has now been approved as a dietary supplement by the FDA. However, for years the FDA had outlawed this sweet food because of their loyalty to Monsanto!

In 1991, the NIH published a bibliography of 167 studies, documenting the adverse effects associated with aspartame,[60] yet thousands of the foods on supermarket shelves still contain this neurotoxic substance. It is known to affect short-term memory[61] and may lead to a wide variety of diseases,[62] including:

- Migraines
- Brain tumors
- Birth defects
- Multiple sclerosis
- Alzheimer's disease
- Diabetes
- Chronic fatigue syndrome
- Epilepsy/seizures
- Fibromyalgia

Very recently, due to an enormous groundswell of resistance to the word "aspartame," Ajinomoto (its current manufacturer) has renamed it to "AminoSweet" and is marketing it as a "natural" product. We again have to urge people who want to be well or get well to always choose organic and fresh foods. These are as safe as possible.

Monosodium Glutamate

This flavor enhancer, developed by a Japanese food chemist in 1907, is tasteless by itself. In its original form, it was a salt derivative of a natural amino acid called glutamate, a common substance found in every plant and animal species. **Eventually, turned into MSG, it found its way into almost every kind of convenience food—from soups, canned gravy, salad dressings, frozen/ready meals to potato chips—and into meals served in the worldwide chains of fast-food restaurants.**

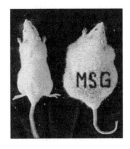

The reason for this lavish use of MSG was discovered by John E. Erb, a research assistant at the University of Waterloo, Ontario, Canada, when he found out that laboratory mice and rats, used for studies on obese animals, had to be injected with MSG soon after birth to make them fat.[63]

Under natural circumstances, no rodents become obese; they only do so when the injected MSG triples the amount of insulin that their pancreas produces. Once fat, they are known as "MSG-treated rats." The awful truth is that MSG is now regularly added to mandated childhood vaccines for the same reason: to predispose the child to future obesity, just as the laboratory rats were.[64]

Away from the research laboratory, MSG is added to human food for its addictive effect. As long ago as 1978, it was scientifically proven to be an addictive substance.[65] Since the food manufacturers' lobby openly states that the purpose of MSG is to make people eat more,[66] this addictive item clearly plays a major role in the current excess weight epidemic.

Huge numbers of people suffer from the serious side effects of MSG, which include headaches, palpitation, vomiting, nausea, numbness, chest pain, drowsiness, facial pressure and weakness.[67] Some of these side effects are also referred to as "Chinese restaurant syndrome."

John E. Erb summed up his findings in *The Slow Poisoning of America*,[68] his book on the harmful activities of the food additive industry. Then Erb checked the cupboards in his kitchen and refrigerator and found that MSG was in everything!

A few examples are Campbell's soups, flavored potato chips from Frito-Lay, Nissin's Top Ramen, Betty Crocker's Hamburger Helper, canned gravy from Heinz, frozen prepared meals from Swanson and salad dressing from Kraft. MSG is also added in abundance to the food at Burger King, McDonald's, Wendy's, Taco Bell and particularly Kentucky Fried Chicken.[69]

Although the dangers of MSG have been widely known for decades, the FDA set no limits on how much of it may be added to foods. They claim that it is "safe" in any amount.[70]

Many people are intolerant of MSG and develop serious allergic symptoms.[71] The problem has been thoroughly studied by Jack I. Samuels and his wife Adrilenne Samuels, PhD. Mr. Samuels is the president and cofounder of the Truth in Labeling Campaign, which was started in 1994. The couple have worked to inform consumers, physicians, researchers and government officials of the dangers of MSG. They have testified at meetings held and/or funded by the FDA and in scientific journals.

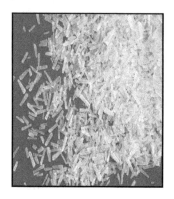

The Samuels have warned the public that it is not easy to identify foods containing MSG due to its acceptance and long-term (grandfathered) use by the FDA.[72] **It is hidden from the public with names such as flavor enhancers, autolyzed yeast, hydrolyzed vegetable protein and textured protein. It also causes increased hunger, cravings, weight gain, water retention, irritability and fatigue.** There are at least 52 different names under which MSG is disguised, since many people now know of its toxicity and read labels to try to avoid it.

MSG is used by scientists to make laboratory animals fat for research purposes. Excess weight will develop in these animals even though they do not increase their food intake![73] MSG appears to affect the hunger/weight control centers of the brain. However, MSG is added to so many foods that, according to the textbook, *Nutritional Biochemistry and Metabolism,* the average American consumes 1.92 pounds of MSG each year. It is addictive and causes people to eat more. That is why the food industry adds it to such a huge number of processed foods.[74]

Here is an abbreviated list of foods that contain MSG:

- Soy sauce
- Canned soups
- Sauces
- Luncheon meats
- Salad dressings
- Dips
- Canned and frozen meats
- Bouillon cubes
- Chicken stock
- Jarred fishes

Here is a list of the hidden names under which MSG masquerades. These ingredients always contain processed free glutamic acid:

- Autolyzed plant protein
- Autolyzed yeast
- Autolyzed yeast extract
- Calcium caseinate
- Calcium glutamate
- Gelatin
- Glutamate
- Glutamic acid
- Anything hydrolyzed, including hydrolyzed plant protein and hydrolyzed vegetable protein
- Magnesium glutamate
- Monoammonium glutamate

- Monopotassium glutamate
- MSG
- Senomix
- Sodium caseinate
- Soy protein
- Soy protein concentrate
- Soy protein isolate
- Textured protein
- Vetsin
- Whey protein
- Whey protein concentrate
- Whey protein isolate
- Yeast extract
- Yeast food
- Yeast nutrient

These ingredients often contain or produce processed free glutamic acid:

- Barley malt
- Bouillon and broth
- Carrageenan (E407)[75]
- Citrate (E330)
- Citric acid
- Anything containing "enzymes"
- Anything "enzyme modified"
- Anything "fermented"
- Any "flavors" or "flavoring"

- Malt extract
- Maltodextrin
- Pectin (E440)
- Protease
- Anything "protein fortified"
- Seasonings
- Stock
- Soy sauce (A reader has informed us that Russell Blaylock, MD, states in his book, *Excitotoxins: The Taste That Kills*, that soy sauce *always* contains MSG.[76])
- Soy sauce extract
- Anything "ultra-pasteurized"

Here are ingredients suspected of containing or creating sufficient processed free glutamic acid that may trigger an MSG-reaction in *highly sensitive* people:

- Brown rice syrup
- Corn starch
- Corn syrup
- Dextrose
- Anything "enriched"
- Lipolyzed butter fat
- Milk powder
- Modified food starch
- Most things "low fat" or "no fat"
- Reduced fat milk (skim, 1% or 2%)
- Rice syrup
- Anything "vitamin enriched"

These work synergistically with MSG to enhance flavor. If they are present for flavoring, so is MSG:

- Disodium 5'-guanylate (E627)

- Disodium 5'-inosinate (E631)

- Disodium 5'-ribonucleotides (E635)

Altered Foods

The only way to exclude these and countless other harmful additives from one's diet is to avoid all manufactured foods; take the more labor-intensive but health-restoring path of eating only fresh, organic natural foods; and limit restaurant meals to rare occasions.

Additive-filled junk food not only harms the body, but is also a powerful trigger for antisocial behavior. Researchers both in California and in England have run experiments in prisons housing young male criminals, giving them supplements containing vitamins, minerals and essential fatty acids over several months, and monitoring their behavior. In both countries, minor offenses dropped by 33%; serious ones, including violence, dropped by 37% to 38%.[77] Take those findings out of the prison setting and it becomes obvious that much antisocial behavior in society can be ascribed directly to harmful toxic food additives—yet another powerful argument for avoiding junk food of all kinds.

Transfats

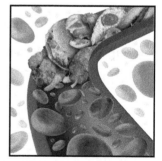

Described variously as the world's unhealthiest food and/or as "heart attack in a box," these ubiquitous food components are produced by hydrogenating vegetable oil to turn a liquid into a solid substance. Transfats or hydrogenated vegetable oils (HVOs) are known to increase the levels of LDL (low-density lipoprotein) or "bad cholesterol," while reducing those of HDL (high-density lipoprotein), the "good" variety. They leave fatty deposits in the arteries, cause digestive disorders and reduce the absorption rate of essential vitamins and minerals.

The Harvard School of Public Health has estimated that at least 30,000 people—probably 100,000—die every year in the United States from cardiovascular disease, caused by eating HVOs found in most convenience foods.[78] The American nutritionist Mary Enig has stated that transfats disrupt the cellular function of the body, weakening its power to expel wastes and toxins.[79] This opens the door to heart disease, diabetes, cancer, poor immunity and excess weight.

The good news is that, since January 2006, under U.S. government regulations, food manufacturers must state the amount of transfats contained in their products.[80] Some have already started to remove transfats from their output. The British Soil Association, flagship of the organic movement in the U.K., has recently declared that all additives, including transfats, MSG and aspartame, are absolutely banned from all organic products[81]—yet another reason to commit ourselves to organic food.

However, the dangers of food additives should not blind us to the fact that the first major culprit of the average modern diet is salt (sodium)—the very substance that's hardest to avoid. Despite official warnings against its overuse,[82] salt consumption in the Western world is alarmingly high. Within the body, it causes water retention, leading to edema and weight gain. Salt also puts an unreasonable burden on the kidneys, raises blood pressure, deadens the taste buds so that more and more is needed to produce an effect, and interferes with the digestive process.

Since meat is a valued staple item of the modern diet, it may sound surprising that excess animal proteins behave as toxins in the body. The fact is that the human organism, with its long intestinal tract, is not designed to cope with a diet high in animal proteins. (By contrast, the intestinal tract of carnivores, such as lions and other big cats, is short—hence the waste products of the digested meat are quickly eliminated.) The ideal diet for humans should be predominantly plant-based, with a minimum of animal proteins[83]; today the opposite applies.

As we go through life, we become less able to digest animal proteins. These poorly digested, incompletely broken down parts linger in the body as toxins. The animal fats contained in almost all meat, poultry and dairy produce are also inadequately digested as the body ages and its enzymes no longer function efficiently. Food animals are raised on unhealthy food treated with hormones, antibi-

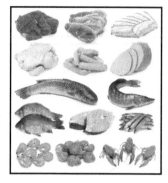

otics and synthetic growth promoters. Whatever they are forced to consume remains in the meat, eggs and milk products that finally land on our tables, adding to the already heavy toxic load we are unwittingly carrying.

The body attempts to get rid of all of these harmful substances to protect itself. Unfortunately, in addition to the massive burden of toxins with which it needs to deal, it also confronts the problem of deficiency.

Fluoride

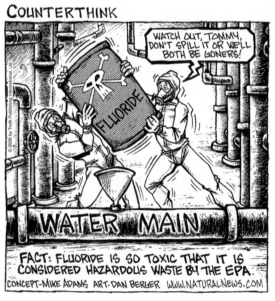

CARTOON CREATED BY MIKE ADAMS (WWW.NATURALNEWS.COM)

Among the factors undermining the body's defenses, fluoride deserves special attention. While exorbitant dental health claims are made for it by commercial interests, **it is in fact a dangerous poison, an industrial waste containing small amounts of lead, mercury, beryllium and arsenic.**[84]

The official reason why the U.S. government promotes the compulsory addition of fluoride to drinking water is to improve children's dental health, which, as common sense recognizes, is not undermined by a shortage of fluoride but by an unhealthy diet, insufficient dental hygiene and too many sweets.

According to some experts,[85] fluoride only protects the teeth of children up to the age of five. Since that age group comprises only a small percentage of the population, it seems indefensible to force this highly controversial chemical onto everybody, irrespective of their age and dental condition. In fact, only 1/2 of 1% of the water in our water supplies is consumed by humans, and only a small fraction of that is consumed by children.[86] The rest of this highly toxic chemical is added to the environment.

Moreover, there is evidence[87] to show that fluoridation does not lastingly improve children's dental health. On the other hand, it causes dental fluorosis in one of every eight children, resulting in mottled, discolored teeth.[88] In the United States, according to figures released in 2003, despite fluoridation, more than half of children aged six to eight years and two-thirds of all 15-year-olds suffer from dental decay.[89] **It is also claimed that the prolonged intake of fluoride can be linked to increased risk of cancers, hip fractures, osteoporosis, kidney trouble and even birth defects.**[90]

The late Dean Burk, MD, who had worked for more than 30 years as chief chemist at the U.S. National Cancer Institute (NCI), declared, "Fluoride causes more human cancer death, and causes it faster, than any other chemical."[91] Following a 17-year study, the NCI found that, as fluoridation increased, so did oral cancer and osteosarcoma, a rare form of bone cancer, in young men.[92]

Despite the NCI study's conclusions, the pro-fluoride camp is doing its utmost to hide and deny the harmful effects of the chemical. One such attempt led to an uproar among scientists in 2006, when it transpired that Professor Chester Douglass of the Harvard Dental School had kept secret the findings of his graduate student Elise B. Bassin for four years. In her 2001 thesis, Bassin discussed the association between fluoride and cancer, particularly osteosarcoma—bone cancer—in young males. When her findings were finally published in May 2006, and the truth came out to general consternation among researchers, **Harvard exonerated Professor Douglass from any wrongdoing and conflict of interest, although he is widely known to be a paid consultant for the toothpaste industry, which is a major user of fluoride.**[93]

Up to 500 letters of protest have been sent to Harvard's President Bok, among them a blistering one from Professor Samuel Epstein, Chairman of the Cancer Prevention Coalition, demanding "a full and watertight explanation of this extraordinary action."[94] At the time of this writing, Professor Douglass is said to have contributed $1 million to the new dentistry building of Harvard[95]—and his crime has thus been "forgiven."

This story is just one of many examples showing how assiduously vested interests fight to protect their profitable products, even at the risk of endangering public health.

Nicotine and Alcohol

The health ravages caused by smoking have been widely known for a long time, yet the habit persists. Smokers use cigarettes either as a stimulant or as an aid to relaxation. In either case, the desired effect wears off quickly and has to be renewed, hence the self-destructive routine of chain smoking.

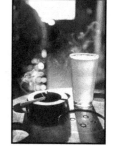

The main active ingredient of tobacco is nicotine, authoritatively described as "one of the most toxic and addictive of all poisons that acts as swiftly as cyanide,"[96] yet nicotine is not the only toxic product of smoking. The tars produced by the burning process line the lungs and eventually cause emphysema and cancer.[97]

Nicotine's bad effects on blood pressure are immediate and severe. Blood cholesterol levels spike up to 100 points higher right after smoking just one cigarette. We leave it to your imagination to visualize the effects of chain smoking, or smoking a pack or two of cigarettes every day.

Smokers tend to assume that they are only damaging their lungs. However, the poisons contained in cigarettes pervade the entire organism, damaging all organs. Bladder cancer, for instance, occurs more frequently among smokers than abstainers.[98] There is also the detrimental effect of the well-documented "second-hand smoke" on the smoker's family and workmates.[99] What may appear to many—even today—as an acceptable social habit is in fact a serious attack on our natural defenses.

The same applies to alcohol, which ideally should only be consumed occasionally and in small amounts. If consumed in excess, alcohol can lead to chronic alcoholism. It is poisonous to the brain and even more so to the liver, and can cause gastritis, pancreatitis, seizures and delirium. In extreme cases, it leads to cirrhosis of the liver and death.[100] Since the liver is a key organ, it is easy to see how its destruction by uncontrolled drinking undermines the entire organism.

Cosmetics

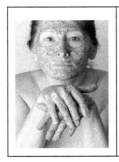 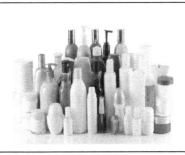 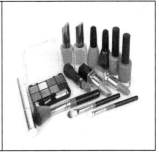

Compared to heavily toxic substances, such as nicotine and alcohol, cosmetics may seem somewhat out of place on our black list. After all, they have been used to enhance beauty and glamour for thousands of years; archeologists have found many remains of precious ointments, lotions and other cosmetics in ancient royal sites and temples.

However, today's cosmetics are vastly different from the natural substances used in ancient Babylon and Egypt. They contain an astounding number of ingredients, many of which (e.g., the wide range of parabens) are toxic. Sodium lauryl sulphate (used in industry to clean garage floors and degrease engines), dioxins (suspected of being carcinogenic) and formaldehyde (a highly irritant toxic substance) are also used. **Since all toxins help to break down the body's defenses, it stands to reason that all sources of toxicity must be eliminated from our daily lives, which includes toxin-rich cosmetics.**

The fact is that up to 60% of all substances sprayed or rubbed into the skin are promptly absorbed and travel straight into the bloodstream. Orthodox medicine makes use of this with the application of various patches, which deliver medications, from painkillers to nicotine to hormone replacements, into the bloodstream. By the same token, powders, creams, ointments, sprays and perfumes also enter the organism fast. (We tell our women patients, "If you wouldn't eat or drink it, don't put it on your skin or lips!" However, we make one tiny concession: eyebrow pencils are permitted.) **The average, makeup-wearing American woman absorbs about five pounds of cosmetic chemicals per year, directly into her bloodstream. If a woman starts wearing cosmetics at age 12 or 13 (and most girls do), by the time she is 33 (20 years later), she will have absorbed about 100 pounds of toxic material contained in cosmetics.**

One of the riskiest "grooming" substances is the underarm deodorant. Almost all brands contain aluminum, which is seriously harmful,[101] especially when we remember that there are many lymph glands in the underarm area that pass on absorbed toxins to the lymphatic system. Even those creams and sticks that are genuinely free from toxic materials and claim to be organic have to be avoided because they interfere with the body's attempt to eliminate poisons by the simple act of perspiration! When the body attempts to detoxify through the sweat glands, the process must not be stopped or hampered.

Blocking the underarm passages with a deodorant will force the toxins back into the lymphatic system around the chest and shoulders and increase the risk of breast cancer—also in men.[102] Since male grooming aids have become widely used, the incidence of male breast cancer has been increasing. We may assume that much of this development is due to men's routine use of underarm deodorants.

So how should we deal with the problem of perspiration? The first rule is to avoid toxic (i.e., nonorganic) foods and drinks so the body doesn't need to work hard to get rid of the residues. Soap and water are the best cleansers. **Healthy perspiration is odorless and requires no chemical weapon to eliminate it.**

Another highly toxic item used by both men and women is the wide range of hair dyes. The scalp is thoroughly "vasculated" (i.e., rich in blood vessels close to the surface), so whatever is put on it gets quickly absorbed into the bloodstream. Most hair dyes are highly toxic.[103] Even the more recent types, containing mainly nontoxic vegetable materials, introduce an alien substance into the organism. This is why **Gerson patients should not use hair dyes of any kind and may only use the mildest shampoos. They are also advised to avoid perfumes, which contain synthetic aromatics, but may use diluted pure glycerin (without rosewater) to smooth dry skin. Men patients in turn have to do without after-shave lotions and aerosol shaving creams.**

Electromagnetic Fields

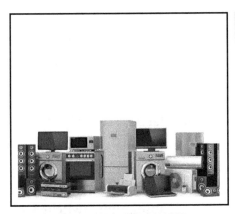

ELECTRICAL APPLIANCES

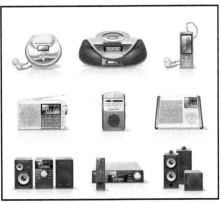

PERSONAL ELECTRONICS

Every living thing is surrounded by its own electromagnetic field—an invisible but measurable layer of radiating energy. For millions of years, these fields existed undisturbed. In the late 19th century, the first incandescent filament light bulb was invented in Britain and then later in America. With that invention, electricity became a vital part of everyday life and its use has grown exponentially.

Today, all populations on Earth are exposed to varying degrees of electromagnetic fields. Lamps, television sets, radios, refrigerators, regular and microwave ovens, computers and latterly "smart" electric and water meters, compact fluorescent lights, wireless computer networks, cellular phones and the millions of cell phone towers all emit invisible electromagnetic frequencies. If we add natural geopathic radiation to our household implements, it is no exaggeration to say that **we exist in an electronic soup or to see that this is bound to have a harmful impact on human health and well-being.**

As the use of cellular phones increases worldwide, more and more radio masts are erected to service them. So far, official bodies have claimed that these masts presented no health risks to people living near them,[104] but concerned individuals tell a different story, reporting on **clusters of diseases, mainly cancer, erupting in the vicinity of a recently erected mast.**[105] **Sleep disturbances, headaches, skin rashes, heart palpitations and vertigo have also set in within the same period.**[106]

Some scientists agree with the concerns of the lay public. For example, Robert O. Becker, MD, twice nominated for the Nobel Prize, called the proliferation of electromagnetic fields "the greatest polluting element in the earth's environment."[107] Both the WHO and the European Parliament have held discussions on the environmental impact of electromagnetic fields.[108]

Applying the precautionary principle, "If in doubt, don't," everything possible must be done to limit the risks of the all-pervasive electronic smog. **Cellular phone use must be cut to a minimum, switched off immediately after use and not carried on the body even when switched off. If possible, hands-free devices should be used to keep phones away from the head and body.**

Lately, the power distribution industry has been virtually forcing homeowners and businesses to install "smart meters." It is extremely important to avoid these devices if at all possible, since they inject "dirty" electricity into the home's electrical system, which then becomes a radiator of electromagnetic radiation. Some people who are particularly sensitive have found their homes to be uninhabitable after the installation of the devices.

Phones aside, **it is wise not to keep any electronic devices, such as clock radios or electronic clocks, near beds where the sleepers would be exposed to radiation throughout the night.** All electronic equipment should be switched off when not in use, not left on stand-by. Some common houseplants (e.g., a Peace Lily) are said to absorb harmful radiation[109] and should be kept in the home in large numbers.

REFERENCES

1. "Protein Damage Through Heating," Innvista. "Protein structure is altered during heating; and, since most people do not eat their meat or eggs raw, this is a major factor to consider." (www.innvista.com/health/nutrition/amino/pdamage.htm).
2. M. Gerson, *A Cancer Therapy, 6th Edition* (San Diego, CA: The Gerson Institute, 2002), p. 175.
3. Personal communication to Charlotte Gerson.
4. U.S. Food and Drug Administration, "Everything Added to Food in the United States (EAFUS)" (www.fda.gov/food/foodingredientspackaging/ucm115326.htm).
5. Lawrence J. Appel, MD, MPH. and Cheryl A. M. Anderson, PhD, MPH, "Compelling Evidence for Public Health Action to Reduce Salt Intake," *New England Journal of Medicine* editorial (10.1056/nejme0910352 nejm.org); "Addressing salt intakes in Europe," FOOD TODAY European Food Information Council, August 2010 (www.eufic.org/article/en/artid/addressing-salt-intakes-in-Europe).
6. C. Gerson and B. Bishop, *Healing the Gerson Way: Defeating Cancer and Other Chronic Diseases, Second Edition* (Carmel, CA: Totality Books, 2009), p. 18.
7. *Taber's Cyclopedic Medical Dictionary, 20th edition* (Philadelphia: F. A. Davis Company, 2005), p. 1175.
8. Note 6 (Gerson), supra, p. 17.

9. M. Dixon and E. C. Webb, *Enzymes (Second Edition)* (New York: Academic Press, 1964), p. 422.

10. T. Colin Campbell, PhD, and Thomas M. Campbell II, MD, *The China Study: Startling Implications for Diet, Weight Loss and Long-term Health* (Dallas: BenBella Books, 2006), p. 58.

11. Note 6 (Gerson), supra, p. 19.

12. Note 7 (*Taber's*), supra, p. 447.

13. Natural Health Restored, "Refined Foods And Processed Foods" (www.natural-health-restored.com/refined-foods.html).

14. "Why is an enzyme destroyed by high temperature?" (http://answers.yahoo.com/question/index?qid=20070704113453AAmUvem).

15. Max Gerson, *A Cancer Therapy: Results of Fifty Cases and The Cure of Advanced Cancer by Diet Therapy: A Summary of Thirty Years of Clinical Experimentation,* 6th ed. (San Diego, CA: Gerson Institute, 2002), p. 176.

16. Ibid., pp. 145-173.

17. B. P. Baker, Charles M. Benbrook, E. Groth III and K. Lutz Benbrook, "Pesticide residues in conventional, integrated pest management (IPM)-grown and organic foods: insights from three US data sets," Taylor and Francis Ltd., *Food Additives and Contaminants* 19 (5) (May 2002): 427-446(20).

18. http://www.naturalnews.com/049120_glyphosate_exposure_WHO_admission_cancer.html

19. Ibid.

20. http://sustainablepulse.com/2015/04/09/monsanto-knew-of-glyphosate-cancer-link-35-years-ago/#.VTGIBJNVGK0

21. http://www.seattleorganicrestaurants.com/vegan-whole-food/toxicity-of-glyphosate-roundup-Monsanto.php

22. Ibid.

23. Ibid.

24. Ibid.

25. http://www.medicaldaily.com/autism-rates-increase-2025-glyphosate-herbicide-may-be-responsible-future-half-316388

26. G. Lean, "Revealed: health fears over secret study into GM food," *The Independent on Sunday* (London) (May 22, 2005).

27. "Chronic" usually means developing slowly, over time, and irreversible or incurable.

28. J. Whitaker, *Dr. Whitaker's Unabridged Dictionary of Drug Alternatives and Non-Surgical Solutions* (Potomac, MD: Healthy Directions, LLC, 2007), pp. 6-10.

29. Gurkirpal Singh, MD, "Recent Considerations in Nonsteroidal Anti-Inflammatory Drug Gastropathy," *The American Journal of Medicine*, July 27, 1998, p. 31S.

30. M. Wolfe, MD, D. Lichtenstein, MD, and Gurkirpal Singh, MD, "Gastrointestinal Toxicity of Nonsteroidal Anti-inflammatory Drugs," *The New England Journal of Medicine,* June 17, 1999, Vol. 340, No. 24, pp. 1888-1889.

31. Brad Case, DC, *Thugs, Drugs and the War on Bugs* (Prunedale, CA: New Renaissance Books, 2010), p. 104.

32. Ibid., p. 104.

33. Note 28 (Whitaker), supra, pp. 6, 7.

34. Note 31 (Case), supra, p. 108.

35. *San Francisco Chronicle*, Jan. 2, 1970.

36. Note 6 (Gerson), supra, p. 120.

37. http://en.wikipedia.org/wiki/Epigenetics.

38. Richard Mackarness, *Eat Fat and Grow Slim* (London: Harvill Press, 1958; London: Fontana/Collins, revised and extended edition, 1975).

39. "The Pew Charitable Trusts' Food Additives Project estimates that there are more than 10,000 chemicals allowed in food that help make this variety possible." Chemicals in Our Food: What We Don't Know May Be Hurting Us, The Pew Charitable Trusts Health Initiative, Apr. 9, 2013 (www.pewhealth.org/other-resource/chemicals-in-our-food-what-we-dont-know-may-be-hurting-us-85899467015).

40. "Aspartame, used by more than 100 million people around the world, is found in more than 6,000 products." Aspartame Fact Sheet, Aspartame Information Center (www.aspartame.org/aspartame-faq/aspartame-fact-sheet/#.Unb6LOI4GAY).

41. "… a few of the published associations in aspartame reactors. They include the initiation or aggravation of diabetes mellitus, hypoglycemia, convulsions, headache, depression, other psychiatric states, hyperthyroidism, hypertension and arthritis; the simulation of multiple sclerosis, Alzheimer's disease and lupus erythematosus; increasing aspartame addiction[12]; an apparent causative role in brain tumors[10]; a neurologic condition in overweight young women known as pseudotumor cerebri; and even the carpal tunnel syndrome.[11]" (www.wnho.net/fdaapprovedepidemic.htm) H. J. Roberts, "Aspartame (NutraSweet) addiction." *Townsend Letter for Doctors & Patients* 2000; 198 (January): 52-57.

42. www.holisticmed.com/aspartame/adverse.txt.

43. Betty Martini, MD, "Aspartame: No Hoax, Crime of the Century (Front Groups in Violation of Title 18, Section 1001 When They Lie About the Aspartame Issue and Stumble Others)" (Duluth, GA), Mission Possible International (Jul. 18, 2004) (www.wnho.net/aspartame_no_hoax.htm).

44. Louis Elsas testifies before Congress. Animals developed brain tumors; *see also* Note 43 (Martini), supra.

45. Ibid.

46. T. Colin Campbell and Thomas M. Campbell II, *The China Study:* Startling Implications for Diet, Weight Loss and Long-term Health (Dallas: BenBella Books, 2005), p. 98.

47. "Aspartame, Decision of the Public Board of Inquiry" (Sept. 30, 1980), Department of Health and Human Services, Food and Drug Administration [Docket number 75F-0355] (www.sweetpoison.com/articles/pdfs/fdapetition.pdf).

48. Aspartame Toxicity Information Center (www.holisticmed.com/aspartame/adverse.txt).

49. James Turner, ESQ, Director of the National Institute of Science, Law, and Public Policy (NISLAPP), *Aspartame/NutraSweet: The History of the Aspartame Controversy* (Washington, DC: National Institute of Science, Law, and Public Policy).

50. "Proven Unsafe But FDA-Approved: Are YOU Still Consuming This Man-Made Poison?" Dr. Joseph Mercola, Aug. 3, 2011. "It is no coincidence that the FDA Chairman who stood in the way of aspartame's approval was removed from office the day Ronald Reagan took office. His replacement was in part orchestrated by Donald Rumsfeld, CEO of G.D. Searle, in order to allegedly get a friendly rubber stamp on the approval of what some doctors have called 'an addictive excitoneurotoxic carcinogenic drug that interacts with drugs and vaccines.'

"But even with a friendly new FDA Chairman in place, the agency still rejected aspartame for approval by a 3-2 margin. What reprehensible, bordering on criminal action did Chairman Hayes do next? He added a sixth member to the approval board, who voted in favor of aspartame. Then, with a 3-3 tie on the issue, Chairman Hayes himself broke the deadlock with his own vote of approval for aspartame.

"So he packed the board and then used his own vote as a tie-breaker. All apparently perfectly legal . . . And one of Hayes' last acts in office before he left the FDA in1983 amid accusations that he was accepting corporate gifts for political favors, was to approve aspartame for use in beverages. Does this sound to you like a man-made synthetic chemical that should have ever been allowed into the world's food supply?" (http://articles.mercola.com/sites/articles/archive/2011/08/03/just-how-bad-is-aspartame.aspx).

51. www.fda.gov/ohrms/dockets/DOCKETS/02p0317/02P-0317_emc-000429-01.pdf (page 2 of 18).

52. www.dorway.com/betty/diabetes.html.

53. J. Roberts, *Aspartame Disease: An Ignored Epidemic* (W. Palm Beach, FL: Sunshine Sentinel Press, 2001). A table in this publication identifies "blindness," "kidney stones," "convulsions" and "grand mal" attacks as symptoms of aspartame poisoning.

54. Congressional Record, Senate, S-5511, May 7, 1985, and part of the protest of the National Soft Drink Association, now American Beverage, is this statement: "Aspartame has been demonstrated to inhibit the carbohydrate-induced synthesis of the neurotransmitter serotonin (Wurtman affidavit). Serotonin blunts the sensation of craving carbohydrates and this is part of the body's feedback system that helps limit consumption of carbohydrate to appropriate levels. Its inhibition by aspartame could lead to the anomalous result of a diet product causing increased consumption of carbohydrates."

55. H. J. Roberts, MD, *Defense Against Alzheimer's Disease* (W. Palm Beach, FL: Sunshine Sentinel Press, April 1995).

56. Ibid.

57. Mary Nash Stoddard, *Deadly Deception: Story of Aspartame: Shocking Expose of the World's Most Controversial Sweetener* (Dallas: Odenwald Press, August 1998). This book also contains the full story and timeline of the campaign to get aspartame approved by the FDA, despite its known dangers. Michael Barbee, *Politically Incorrect Nutrition: Finding Reality in the Mire of Food Industry Propaganda* (Ridgefield, CT: Vital Health Publishing, April 2004). In this book, Barbee quotes Dr. Louis Elias, Pediatric Professor in Genetics at Emory University.

58. A resident of Marietta, Georgia, "Dr. Joe" is the president of Health Plus Wellness Center, a multidisciplinary health care center specializing in preventive health care and life extension. He is also the author of *Eating Right* (www.rense.com/health/sweetners.htm).

59. D. Gates, "The FDA and Stevia"; [Internet]. Bogart (GA): Body Ecology; 2010 [cited May 15, 2010]. Available from: www.stevia.net/fda.htm. Note: the Stevia site is part of the Body Ecology site (www.bodyecology.com). FDA statement that there is no basis to object to the use of certain refined Stevia preparations: www.fda.gov/AboutFDA/Basics/ucm194320.htm.

Stevia Import Alert from FDA site: www.accessdata.fda.gov/cms_ia/importalert_119.html.

60. U.S. National Institutes of Health, "Adverse Effects of Aspartame: January '86 through December '90" (1991), a bibliography of 167 studies documenting adverse effects associated with aspartame.

61. www.dorway.com/92symptomsfotocopy.html.

62. Ibid.

63. John E. and T. M. Erb, *The Slow Poisoning of America* (available on-line at https://www.spofamerica.com).

64. "Monosodium glutamate (MSG) and 2-phenoxy-ethanol which are used as stabilizers in a few vaccines to help the vaccine remain unchanged when the vaccine is exposed to heat, light, acidity, or humidity." Ingredients of Vaccines – Fact Sheet, Centers for Disease Control and Prevention (www.cdc.gov/vaccines/vac-gen/additives.htm).

65. Note 63 (Erb), supra.

66. Ibid.

67. www.dorway.com/92symptomsfotocopy.html.

68. Note 63 (Erb), supra.

69. Burger King (www.bk.com/cms/en/us/cms_out/digital_assets/files/pages/IngredientsDeclaration.pdf); McDonald's (nutrition.mcdonalds.com/nutritionexchange/ingredientslist.pdf); Wendy's (http://wendys.com/food/pdf/us/nutrition.pdf); Taco Bell (www.tacobell.com/nutrition/ingredient-statement); Kentucky Fried Chicken (www.kfc.com/nutrition/pdf/kfc_ingredients_may10.pdf).

70. As quoted from herbsspices, Monday (4/12/2010), the FDA acknowledge MSG as safe a product as salt, pepper and sugar (http://medicmagic.net/how-safe-is-msg-to-consume.html#more-4049).

71. www.truthinlabeling.org/I.AreYouSensitive.html.

72. www.truthinlabeling.com/SomethingToThinkAbout.html.

73. www.ncbi.nlm.nih.gov/pubmed/3785512?dopt=Abstract&holding=npg.

74. "Q: What is MSG and what is the problem with it? A: MSG stands for monosodium glutamate, a substance extracted from grains or beets. In the Eastern world it is referred to as the 'magic powder of the East.' We won't bore you with it's [sic] chemical properties. There is great variation in how much MSG can be found in foods, but according to the textbook— NUTRITIONAL BIOCHEMISTRY AND METABOLISM—the average American consumes 1.92 pounds of MSG each year." (www.carbohydrateaddicts.com/msg.html).

75. Russell Blaylock, *Excitotoxins: the Taste That Kills* (Albuquerque: Health Press, 1996).

76. Ibid.

77. B. Gesch, London press conference, Royal College of Psychiatrists (Jun. 25, 2002); S. Schoenthaler, *Anti-Ageing Medical Publications,* Vol. III. (Marina del Rey, CA: Health Quest Publications, 1999).

78. D. Mozaffarian, et al., "Trans Fatty Acids and Cardiovascular Disease," *New England Journal of Medicine* 15 (354) (Apr. 13, 2006): 1601-1613; *see also* "Trans Fatty Acids and Coronary Heart Disease" ("In an updated analysis of the trans fat-heart disease link, HSPH researchers have found that removing trans fats from the industrial food supply could prevent tens of thousands of heart attacks and cardiac deaths each year in the U.S. The findings are published in the April 13, 2006 issue of the New England Journal of Medicine. . . . Trans fats have also been associated with an increased risk of coronary heart disease in epidemiologic studies. . . . Based on the available metabolic studies, we estimated in a 1994 report that approximately 30,000 premature coronary heart disease deaths annually could be attributable to consumption of trans fatty acids.[4]" Note 4: W. C. Willett, A. Ascherio, "Trans fatty acids: Are the effects only marginal?," *Am J Public Health* 1994; 84: 722-724.) (www.hsph.harvard.edu/reviews/transfats.html)

79. Interview with Richard A. Passwater, "Health Risks from Processed Foods and the Dangers of Trans Fats."

80. "Food Labeling: Trans Fatty Acids in Nutrition Labeling . . ." U.S. Department of Health and Human Services, FDA 21 CFR Part 101, Federal Register (Jul. 11, 2003), p. 41434.

81. "What we can say—the quality and benefits of organic food," British Soil Association information sheet, Version 4 (Nov. 24, 2005).

82. "Excessive Sodium is One of the Greatest Health Threats in Foods," World Health Organization (WHO) report from October 2006 meeting in Paris, part of the implementation of the WHO's Global Strategy on Diet, Physical Activity and Health.

83. Emma Young, "Trace arsenic in water raises cancer risk," *New Scientist* (Sept. 14, 2001).

84. J. A. Brunette and J. P. Carlos, "Recent Trends in Dental Caries in U.S. Children and the Effect of Water Fluoridation," *Journal of Dental Research* 69 (Spec. Issue February 1990): 723-727.

85. Ibid.

86. "Fluoride—intended only for human consumption by people under 14 years of age—is injected into our drinking water supply at approximately 1 part-per-million (ppm), but since we only drink 1/2 of one percent of the total water supply, the rest literally goes down the drain as a free hazardous-waste disposal for the chemical industry, where we PAY them so that we can flush their expensive hazardous waste down our toilets." Fluoride—The Lunatic Drug," Shirley Carroll, American Patriot Friends Network. Aug. 13, 2000.

87. M. A. Awad, J. A. Hargreaves, and G. W. Thompson, "Dental Caries and Fluorosis in 7-9 and 11-14 Year Old Children Who Received Fluoride Supplements from Birth," *Journal of the Canadian Dental Association* 60 (4) (1991): 318-322.

88. C. H. Shiboski, et al., "The association of early childhood caries and race/ethnicity among California preschool children," *Journal of Public Health Dentistry* 63 (1) (2003): 38-46.

89. Elise B. Bassin, D. Wypij, R. B. Davis and M. A. Mittleman, "Age-specific fluoride exposure in drinking water and osteosarcoma (United States)," *Cancer Causes and Control* 17 (2006): 421-428.

90. John Yiamouyiannis, PhD, "Fluoride, the Silent Killer" (www.consumerhealth.org/articles/display.cfm?ID=19990303222823).

91. Dean Burk, MD, Congressional Record (Jul. 21, 1976).

92. Perry D. Cohn, "A Brief Report on the Association of Drinking Water Fluoridation and the Incidence of Osteosarcoma Among Young Males," Environmental Health Service, New Jersey Department of Health (Nov. 8, 1992). In 1992, the New Jersey State Department of Health released the results of a study which found six times more bone cancer among males under the age of 20 living in communities with fluoridated water.

93. Juliet Eilperin, "Professor at Harvard Is Being Investigated, Fluoride-Cancer Link May Have Been Hidden," *The Washington Post* (Jul. 13, 2005), p. A03.

94. Letter from Professor Samuel Epstein to Harvard University President Derek C. Bok (Aug. 31, 2006).

95. "Douglass' donation of around $1 million to Harvard in 2001 also came to light, sparking debate over the propriety of a school conducting an investigation against a major donor." A. Haven Thompson, "At the Harvard School of Dental Medicine, One Professor's Fluoride Scandal Stinks," *The Harvard Crimson*. Sep. 27, 2006 (www.thecrimson.com/article/2006/9/27/at-the-harvard-school-of-dental/).

96. *Taber's Cyclopedic Medical Dictionary* (Philadelphia: F. A. Davis Company, 2005).

97. "Questions About Smoking, Tobacco, and Health," American Cancer Society (www.cancer.org/docroot/PED/content/PED_10_2x_Questions_About_Smoking_Tobacco_and_Health.asp).

98. "Detailed Guide: Bladder Cancer, What Are the Risk Factors for Bladder Cancer?," American Cancer Society (www.cancer.org/docroot/cri/content/cri_2_4_2x_what_are_the_risk_factors_for_bladder_cancer_44.asp).

99. "Secondhand Smoke—It Takes Your Breath Away: Secondhand Smoke is unhealthy . . ." New York State Department of Health (www.health.state.ny.us/prevention/tobacco_control/second/second.htm).

100. Howard J. Worman, MD, "Alcoholic Liver Disease," Columbia University Department of Medicine (http://cpmcnet.columbia.edu/dept/gi/alcohol.html).

101. M. S. Petrik, M. C. Wong, R. C. Tabata, R. F. Garry and C. A. Shaw, "Aluminum adjuvant linked to gulf war illness induces motor neuron death in mice," *Neuromolecular Medicine* 9 (1) (2007): 83-100.

102. P. D. Darbre, et al., "Chemical Used in Deodorant Found in Breast Cancer Tissue," *Journal of Applied Toxicology* 24 (1) (2004).

103. F. N. Marzulli, S. Green and H. K. Haibach, "Hair dye toxicity—a review," *Journal of Environmental Pathology, Toxicology and Oncology* 1 (4) (March-April 1978): 509-30.

104. "Cell Phone Facts: Consumer Information on Wireless Phones," U.S. Food and Drug Administration (www.fda.gov/cellphones/qa.html#4).

105. "Cancer clusters at phone masts," *The London Sunday Times* (Apr. 22, 2007).

106. Eileen O'Connor, "EMF Discussion Group at the Health Protection Agency for Radiation Protection (HPA-RPD) on 2nd March 2006" (October 2006), Mobile Phone/Mast Radiation (www.mast-victims.org/index.php?content=journal&action=view&type=journal&id=111).

"Six other short-term mobile phone mast studies have also found significant health effects such as headaches, dizziness, depression, fatigue, sleep disorder, difficulty in concentration and cardiovascular problems:

"1) H-P Hutter, H Moshammer, P Wallner and M Kundi (http://oem.bmjjournals.com/cgi/content/abstract/63/5/307) Subjective symptoms, sleeping problems, and cognitive performance in subjects living near mobile phone base stations: Conclusion: Despite very low exposure to HF-EMF, effects on wellbeing and performance cannot be ruled out, as shown by recently obtained experimental results; however, mechanisms of action at these low levels are unknown. . . .

"2) Santini et al (Paris) [Pathologie Biologie (Paris)] 2002 (http://www.emrnetwork.org/position/santini_hearing march6_02.pdf)

"3) Netherlands Ministries of Economic Affairs, Housing, Spatial Planning and Environment and Health Welfare and Sport. (TNO) 2003 (http://www.unizh.ch/phar/sleep/handy/tnoabstractE.htm)

"4) The Microwave Syndrome – Further Aspect of a Spanish Study – Oberfeld Gerd. Press International Conference in Kos (Greece), 2004 (www.mindfully.org/Technology/2004/Microwave-Syndrome-Oberfeld1may04.htm)

"5) Austrian scientists Dr Gerd Oberfeld send out a press release 1 May 2005 with this report: 'A study in Austria examined radiation from a mobile phone mast at a distance of 80 metres; EEG tests of 12 electro-sensitive people proved significant changes in the electrical currents of the brains. Volunteers for the test reported symptoms like buzzing in the head, palpitations of the heart, un-wellness, light headedness, anxiety, breathlessness, respiratory problems, nervousness, agitation, headache, tinnitus, heat sensation and depression.

"6) Bamberg, Germany 26-April, 2005 Dr C Waldmann-Selsam, Dr U. Säeger, Bamberg, Oberfranken evaluated the medical complaints of 356 people who have had long-term [radiation] exposure in their homes from pulsed high frequency magnetic fields (from mobile phone base stations, from cord-less DECT telephones, amongst others)." *See also* Warren Brodey, MD, "Radiation and Health," Oslo, Norway (Sept. 13, 2006), p. 14 (www.computer-clear.com/radiation_and_health.pdf).

107. Linda Moulton Howe, "British Cell Phone Safety Alert and An Interview with Robert O. Becker, MD," Council on Wireless Technology Impacts (www.energyfields.org/science/becker.html).

108. "Minutes of the Seventh International Advisory Committee Meeting," The International EMF Project (Geneva), World Health Organization (Jun. 6-7, 2002) (www.who.int/peh-emf/publications/IAC_minutes_2002MR_update.pdf).

109. Mary Lambert, *Clearing the Clutter for Good Feng Shui* (New York: Michael Friedman Publishing Group, Jan. 1, 2001). Lambert suggests that the following plants are especially good for absorbing electromagnetic emissions from computers and other electronics: Peace Lily, Peperomias, Cirrus peruvianus (a cactus) and Dwarf Banana Plants. Studies conducted by the National Aeronautics and Space Administration have shown it to be particularly effective in absorbing formaldehyde, xylene, benzene and carbon monoxide from the air in homes or offices.

PART III

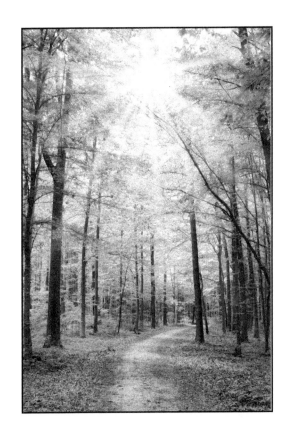

The Path to Healing

CHAPTER 10

Epigenetics: The "New" Science

As is so often the case, "new discoveries in science" are old beliefs, investigated with modern methods, and found correct! One such topic is now called "epigenetics." There have already been some 20 years of intensive study of this "new science." **The prefix "epi" comes from a Greek word meaning "above"; in other words, the news is that there is something *above* genes that can change them.** For decades, we have been made to believe that the Darwinian DNA (deoxyribonucleic acid), or gene theory, was cast in concrete; however, **it turns out that genes can be influenced, silenced or newly activated!**[1]

In 1809, some 50 years before Charles Darwin published his *On the Origin of Species*, French naturalist, Jean-Baptiste Larmarck, wrote about his own theory of evolution. He felt that characteristics acquired during an individual's lifetime can be passed on to his offspring. The idea did not survive Darwin and Gregor Mendel's discovery of genetics.

Their work stood fast, and genes were considered firm and unchangeable; however, that idea has changed. Through recent research, it has become increasingly clear that environmental factors, such as diet and stress, have biological consequences that can be transmitted to offspring without change to the gene sequence. This is a whole new way of looking at genetics and has been dubbed the "new Lamarckism."[2]

Robyn Ward of the Lowy Cancer Research Centre at the University of New South Wales in Sydney, Australia, feels that this is a new way of looking at the inheritance and causes of various diseases, including schizophrenia, bipolar disorder, diabetes and cancer.[3]

The clearest example comes from honeybees. All female honeybees develop from genetically identical larvae, but those fed on royal jelly become fertile queens, while the rest remain sterile workers![4]

A research team, led by Ryszard Maleszka at the Australian National University in Canberra, showed that an epigenetic mechanism accounts for this. His team used RNAi, an enzyme needed for adding the methyl group to DNA in honeybee larvae. Most of these larvae emerged as queens without having been given royal jelly.[5]

In 2000, Randy Jirtle, at Duke University in Durham, North Carolina, led a very important experiment on a strain of genetically identical mice. These carried the *agouti* gene, which makes them fat and prone to diabetes and cancer. Jirtle and his student, Robert Waterland, gave one group of females a diet rich in the methyl groups (folates, green leaves and B_{12}) before conception and during pregnancy. They found that the offspring were very different from their parents. They were slim and lived to a ripe old age. They did contain the *agouti* gene but the methyl groups had superseded its expression![6]

In 2006, Tony Hsiu-Hai Chen, at the National Taiwan University in Taipei, and his colleagues reported that the offspring of men who regularly chewed betel nuts had twice the normal risk of developing "metabolic syndrome" (the new name for a combination of obesity, diabetes and high blood pressure) during childhood.[7] Betel nuts are also associated with several symptoms of metabolic syndrome in chewers including increased heart rate, blood pressure, waist size and body weight.[8]

There is even evidence that epigenetic changes can affect mate preference. Last year, David Crews and Andrea Gore, at the University of Texas at Austin, published a study of male rats whose great-grandfathers had been exposed to the fungicide vinclozolin. Previous research has revealed that such exposure leads to increased infertility and higher risks of cancer even four generations later. Crews and Gore found that female rats tended to avoid these males. They could sense something was wrong, says Gore. She adds that the females seemed to select mates on the basis of an epigenetic pattern, as opposed to a genetic difference.[9]

In 2010, the NIH will invest more than $190 million over the next five years to accelerate an emerging field of biomedical research known as epigenomics.[10] The list of illnesses to be studied in the resulting grants reveals the scope of this emerging field including cancer, Alzheimer's disease, autism, schizophrenia, asthma, kidney disease, glaucoma and muscular dystrophy. All these problems—supposedly "incurable" or "genetic"—have already been cured by the Gerson Therapy![11]

As we have seen in previous articles, the reports of autism being caused by vaccinations are numerous and disturbing.[12] However, autism has also been reversed by intensive detoxification by the Gerson Therapy,[13] or other similar methods.[14]

Here is a case that illustrates epigenetics both ways: Faye, at age 12, was suffering from advanced cystic fibrosis, and constant and continuing infections and mucous discharge into her lungs. This problem was treated by orthodox medicine with the usual antibiotics, which never cure. The girl had chest pain, breathing difficulties, was not growing or developing normally and her disease was characterized as "genetic." This gives the orthodox physicians an excuse for saying it is "incurable" but clearly not their fault! People with the disease do not usually survive past the age of 21 or 22.

The case had two points, as indicated above. The child was born apparently normal and healthy. At the age of six months, she was vaccinated with diphtheria, pertussis and tetanus. This started her problems—possibly a toxic aggravation of some dormant genes.

When she started the Gerson Therapy, her constant infections, gummed-up lungs, pain and delayed development all disappeared. She developed normally and needed no further antibiotics. With the excellent fresh and green nutrients, apparently the aforementioned "methylation" that the therapy provides, contrary to all forecasts, and the usual prognosis of this disease, she was able to get married and have a healthy baby! Now, past the age of 30, she is alive and well.

REFERENCES

1. C. Gerson, "The 'new' science of epigenetics," *Gerson Healing Newsletter,* March-April 2010. p. 6.
2. "Newsweek: Transgenerational epigenetics is 'the new Lamarckism.'" "A recent article in Newsweek from science writer Sharon Begley reports on 'the new Lamarckism,' citing studies from epigenetics researchers, including Emma Whitelaw. The article seems to be all about transgenerational epigenetics, but rather than ever use the word 'epigenetics,' the favored term is 'the new Lamarckism.'" *Epigenetic News,* Jan 26, 2009.
3. M. P. Hitchins and R. L. Ward, "Favoritism in DNA Methylation," *Cancer Prev Res,* October 2009 2; 847.
4. Vinod K. Wadhawan, "COMPLEXITY EXPLAINED: 2. Swarm Intelligence," 22 August 2009. "It may be mentioned here that all female honeybees, including the queen bees, develop from larvae which are identical genetically. Those fed on a certain 'royal jelly' become fertile queens, while the rest remain sterile workers." (http://nirmukta.com/2009/08/22/complexity-explained-2-swarm-intelligence/).
5. S. Foret, R. Kucharski, Y. Pittelkow, G. A. Lockett and R. Maleszka, "Epigenetic regulation of the honey bee transcriptome: unravelling the nature of methylated genes," *BMC Genomics,* 10:472, Oct. 14, 2009.
6. E. Watters, "DNA Is Not Destiny: The new science of epigenetics rewrites the rules of disease, heredity, and identity," *Discover Magazine,* Nov. 2006.
7. Fu-Mei Chung, Dao-Ming Chang, Miao-Pei Chen, Jack C. R. Tsai, Yi-Hsin Yang, Tien-Yu Shieh, Shyi-Jang Shin, MD, Tony Hsiu-Hsi Chen, Tong-Yuan Tai and Yau-Jiunn Lee, "Areca Nut Chewing Is Associated With Metabolic Syndrome: Role of tumor necrosis factor-?, leptin, and white blood cell count in betel nut chewing-related metabolic derangements," *Diabetes Care,* July 2006, Vol. 29 No. 7, p. 1714.
8. Emma Young, "Rewriting Darwin: The new non-genetic inheritance," *New Scientist* magazine, Issue 2664, 9 July 2008, pp. 28-33.
9. Note 8 (Young), supra.
10. "NIH Announces New Initiative in Epigenomics," *NIH News,* National Institutes of Health, Jan. 22, 2008.
11. M. Gerson, *A Cancer Therapy: Results of Fifty Cases and The Cure of Advanced Cancer by Diet Therapy: A Summary of Thirty Years of Clinical Experimentation,* 6th ed. (San Diego, CA: Gerson Institute, 1999); C. Gerson, "Alzheimer's Disease," *Gerson Healing Newsletter,* Vol. 25, No. 5, Sep.–Oct. 2010, p. 5; C. Gerson, *Asthma: Healing Lung Cancer and*

Respiratory Diseases (Carmel, CA: Totality Books, 2002), p. 12; C. Gerson, "Autism," *Gerson Healing Newsletter*, Vol. 22, No. 2, Mar.–Apr. 2007, p. 7; C. Gerson, "Glaucoma," *Gerson Healing Newsletter*, Vol. 21, No. 2, Mar.–Apr. 2006, p. 6; C. Gerson, "Kidney Disease," *Gerson Healing Newsletter*, Vol. 17, No. 4, Jul.–Aug. 2002, p. 6.

12. "Autism Spectrum Disorders" (www.health-reports.com/autism.html).

13. C. Gerson, "Good News About Autism," *Gerson Healing Newsletter*, Vol. 22, No. 2, Mar.–Apr. 2007, p. 7.

14. "Reverse Autism" (www.squidoo.com/reverse-autism).

CHAPTER 11

Restoring the Healing Mechanism

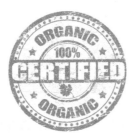

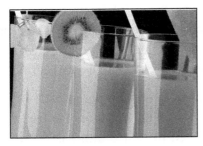
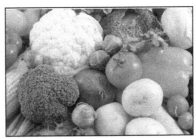

I look forward optimistically to a healthy, happy world as soon as its children are taught the principles of simple and rational living. We must return to nature and nature's God.

—*Luther Burbank (1849–1926)*

> Physicians and the public have exclusively focused on drug therapy to the detriment of at least one of the foundations of good health—appropriate nutrition.
>
> —*Dr. Mary Keith, St. Michael's Hospital,*
> *Toronto, Ontario*

D r. Max Gerson called the body's defenses its "healing mechanism." He repeatedly observed in his patients that this vital defense had degenerated into a diseased state.

As we have seen, two major problems are present in chronic disease: toxicity and nutritional deficiency. If we recognize this fact, we can overcome them both: deficiency through hyperalimentation (the administration of an amount of nutrients that exceeds the appetite) and toxicity through detoxification.

Hyperalimentation

Seriously ill patients are usually unable to eat much. They have a poor appetite, poor digestion and inadequate elimination. Therefore, Dr. Gerson found that juicing was the answer to providing active nutrients.

Almost every patient is able to drink a freshly prepared glass of juice every hour. In a very few cases, for the first few days on the treatment, the usual hourly 8-ounce glass is reduced to 4 or 6 ounces. Using vitamin and mineral pills doesn't work, since the sick body is unable to assimilate pharmaceutically prepared substances. It accepts only juices and foods freshly prepared from living, raw vegetables and fruit. Surprisingly, after only a few days of juicing, potassium supplementation and intensive detoxifying, the patients are able to eat three full vegetarian meals prepared from fresh, organic produce. Once the normal intake of 10-13 glasses of juice plus three full meals and fruit snacks is achieved, the patients are actually able to ingest nutrient value from approximately 20 pounds of fresh foods a day. This achieves the needed hyperalimentation.

The juices are freshly prepared, exclusively from organic fruits and vegetables. For the patient suffering from cancer or other serious chronic disease, the juices are as follows:

- 1 glass of orange juice, or grapefruit juice for diabetes patients (at breakfast)

- 5 glasses of a 50/50 mixture of apples and carrots (for patients with high blood sugar, green juices are substituted for 2-3 apple/carrot juices)

- 4 glasses of "green" juices made from lettuce, chard, red cabbage, green pepper and apple

- 3 glasses of straight carrot juice

Of course, there is a reason for the variation in the juices. People assume that citrus is used to supply vitamin C, and indeed the orange or grapefruit juice does contain it; however, other juices are even richer in that important vitamin!

Carrots are extremely rich in numerous minerals and vegetarian protein. The apples in the mixed juice are high in potassium. Apples in the green juices are high in pectin, which makes these juices more easily digestible.

The "green" juice contains a high level of oxidizing enzymes needed to supply the blood with oxygen—another defense against disease as well as germs and viruses. This juice must be consumed immediately and not be stored since it rapidly loses its enzymes.

The juices are adjusted for some patients (e.g., diabetics, who are given less apple/carrot juice and more "green" juice until their blood sugar stabilizes). In case of diarrhea, two ounces of oatmeal gruel are added to the juices to make them more easily digestible (see Chapter 20, "Understanding Healing Reactions," p. 171).

Meals

For the typical average daily menu of the Gerson patient, see Chapter 17, "Preparing Food and Juices —The Basic Rules," then "The Daily

Routine," p. 150. The particular combination of vegetables used in the "Special Soup or Hippocrates Soup" (see "Special Soup or Hippocrates Soup," p. 152) is specifically used to clear toxins from the kidneys. These vegetables play a major role in detoxifying the body and are helped by the juices and the soup. Other components of the therapy work toward cleansing and detoxifying the liver.

Note that most people are used to the average diet, which invariably contains a lot of sodium. As a result, their taste buds are deadened and, during the first week or so of the treatment, the salt-free Gerson diet tastes "flat" or even "like straw." During that time, patients are urged to use a lot of raw garlic (which should be provided, along with a garlic press) to flavor soup, vegetables, the salad dressing and potatoes. In a few days, the excess sodium is excreted, the taste buds recover and the patients begin to taste and enjoy the food. Actually, the organic produce (correctly prepared instead of boiled in water) is tastier than the commercially grown vegetables. The patients can tell the difference and rarely want to go back to nonorganic foods.

Midday Rest or Sleep

Healing requires energy. Rest is crucial, so the body can use its still-limited energy for healing. The patient is urged to have at least an hour of total rest after lunch, without watching television or reading; a nap would be most beneficial. A diabetic and/or obese patient should also make room for two to three short walks. He or she should also aim to go to sleep shortly after 10 pm, without watching television or reading. Prayer and/or meditation or some gentle (classical) music can be very soothing and promote peace of mind, sound sleep and healing.

In the early days of the Gerson treatment, the body excretes large amounts of sodium. This can cause the patient to wake up during the night, feeling very thirsty. Since no juice will be available and drinking water is discouraged, the patient should be provided with a thermos of peppermint tea. The argument that tea is essentially water doesn't hold. Peppermint tea helps digestion and promotes the production of stomach acid, while plain water dilutes the already low stomach acid of patients suffering from chronic disease. Beside peppermint tea, chamomile tea is suggested for its calming effect, while valerian tea helps to induce sleep.

Detoxification

It is extremely important to understand that, when the body is being flooded with living nutrients, these readily enter the tissues. At that point, they force the accumulated toxins out of the cells and into the bloodstream. In the course of years of eating the average diet, one cannot help but ingest and accumulate high levels of food additives, residues of pesticides and other toxins that block the normal functions of the liver. Thus, the liver becomes unable to release the extra toxins eliminated from the tissues now being flooded with living nutrients.

The Gerson treatment, using the rapidly detoxifying coffee enemas, clears this problem. It is critical to take this detoxification seriously in order to avoid overloading the liver with excreted poisons. Without the coffee enemas, the additional load of toxins released and flooding the system could poison the liver.

Please note: Do not apply the Gerson Therapy unless coffee enemas are included. (See Chapter 18, "All About Enemas," p. 155.)

Medication

The Gerson Therapy also includes several items of medication (see Chapter 21, "The Gerson Therapy for Nonmalignant Diseases," Table 21-1, "Schedule for Nonmalignant Patients," p. 178). These are not synthetic drugs aiming to suppress pain or stimulate some organ. They mainly consist of nutrients or substances that the body is not able to produce in its state of deficiency.

Potassium

Dr. Gerson found that the chronically ill patient was severely depleted of potassium. This allowed sodium to invade the cells and cause great damage. While fresh vegetables and especially fruit are high in potassium, it takes a good deal of additional supplementation to restore this essential mineral to the body.

Pancreatin

Pancreatic enzymes are vital for the digestion of foods. They recognize and are able to digest foreign proteins and therefore play an important role in breaking down arterial plaque (atherosclerosis).

Thyroid and Iodine (Lugol's Solution)

These are given to help the thyroid gland to produce the thyroid hormone, which controls the metabolism as well as the body's heat production, including fever, and by extension the immune system. The nonsynthetic thyroid supplement, extracted from animal thyroid, and the iodine (Lugol's solution at half strength) are used until the metabolism reaches normal levels.

Niacin (Nicotinic Acid, or Vitamin B₃)

Dr. Gerson states[1] that niacin helps to restore sufficient glycogen to the liver, aids in the protein metabolism and acts to open small arteries and capillaries for improved circulation. While doing this, it often causes the well-known "niacin flush"—the dilation of capillaries that causes redness and mild itching in the area above the chest. This flush can alarm the patient, yet it is totally harmless and usually ceases after the first week or two on the Gerson Therapy. Those who find it annoying are advised to let the tiny (50 mg) niacin tablet melt under their tongue.

Warning: So-called "flush free" or "nonflush" niacin is generally niacinamide and, as such, is useless. Please do not use it. *Niacin does not cause bleeding*; however, if bleeding is present (including during menstruation), niacin should be discontinued.

Liver Injection with Vitamin B$_{12}$

Since the healing activity is centered in the liver, and since the liver is toxic and severely damaged, Dr. Gerson used every possible means to help its restoration. The liver extract (3 cc) with additional B$_{12}$ (1/10th cc), given daily, supply substances to help restore the liver as well as the bone marrow. The bone marrow produces red blood cells (for oxygen transport throughout the body), white blood cells (which protect the body from foreign invaders) and platelets (needed for forming blood clots to stop bleeding). The injections (see "Instructions for Giving Injections[2]," p. 107) are given intramuscularly, somewhat behind the hip bone. Dr. Gerson instructed nurses to administer these shots into the "gluteus medius" where it is better absorbed—not the "maximus," which is usually selected, since liver extract is not well assimilated in the fatty tissue of this muscle. Daily shots are given on alternate sides of the body.

Patients are surprised that vitamin C is not supplemented. The reason is that the fresh juices supply this vitamin in very ample amounts, making the pharmaceutical variety unnecessary. Vitamin B$_{12}$ is given to aid in the production of iron-rich red blood cells.

Instructions for Giving Injections[2]

When you return home, you will probably be administering your own injections. During your stay at the Gerson Therapy Center, injections are administered by your medical staff. Learn how to give your own injections by observing, experiencing and asking questions.

1.   Assemble items needed:

   - Alcohol

   - Cotton

   - Syringe

- Extra needle

- Crude liver extract

- Vitamin B_{12}

2. Bottle: Remove protective metal covers from rubber stopper.

3. With alcohol swab, clean tops of bottles.

4. Keep needle and syringe sterile (do not touch).

5. Turn B_{12} bottle upside down and push syringe needle through stopper. Pull out 0.1 cc (just a few drops) to the first small line on the barrel of syringe. Withdraw needle from B_{12}. Draw 3 cc of air into syringe. Turn crude liver bottle upside down and push needle up through center of stopper. Keeping liver extract bottle in an upside-down position, push some air into crude liver bottle and pull some liver extract out, repeating this process until you have pulled out 3 cc of liver extract (pull plunger to first line below 3 cc marking to allow for B_{12}).

6. Remove and discard needle. It is now too dull for injection use.

7. Screw new needle into syringe. (Use 25-gauge 5/8- or 1-inch needle.) Gently tap the side of syringe to gather bubbles to the top of syringe. When bubbles are gathered, press plunger until a tiny bit of fluid spurts from needle. Syringe is now ready to be used. (Put needle cover on loosely.)

8. Clean injection area well with alcohol and cotton.

Locating injection area: Locate the ridge of your hipbone (iliac crest) where your side pants seam runs, roughly in the middle of your side. Measure down the width of two fingers and back 1 inch. That is where the needle goes. The needle should go through the fatty tissue into the muscle. Alternate sides with each injection.

**Hanson's Modification of
Classic Method of Locating
Upper Outer Quadrant**

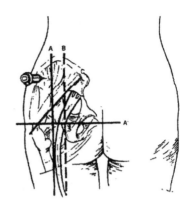

9. Spread skin and push needle in.

10. Push plunger down slowly.

11. Pull needle out and rub area with alcohol for 30 seconds. If bleeding occurs, press cotton to wound. It will stop bleeding very shortly.

12. Break needle and disassemble syringe. Keep broken needles in small cardboard box. Tape box shut when full and discard.

13. Clean open liver and B_{12} bottles with alcohol and store in refrigerator. Protect with fresh baggie after each use. Store unopened liver extract bottles in refrigerator.

Exercise

When the Gerson Therapy is dealing with advanced conditions, the patients have to be warned that healing requires energy and therefore rest; however, problems with obesity, diabetes and sometimes even high blood pressure benefit from exercise.

It is always unwise to overdo, yet with obese patients mild exercise is desirable. Obviously, it will help toward weight loss and improved circulation. In the case of diabetes, it also helps to burn excess sugar and thus activate healing.

If the patient is very ill, weak, or has poor muscle control and/or very poor circulation with possible pain in the extremities, it is clear that exercise will have to wait until pain, lack of control and especially high blood pressure clear up with the organic, salt-free food, juices, enemas and appropriate supplements. The wait is usually not long! The therapy works amazingly fast and severe symptoms disappear. Still, one must not force this issue.

The "Triad"

In many cases, Dr. Gerson used these three tablets to great effect. Once the patient is sufficiently detoxified, they act more powerfully together than they would separately. The "triad," as we call this combination, continues to be effective for pain relief as well as helping promote sound sleep.

The pain triad consists of one regular aspirin (325 mg), one 500 mg tablet of vitamin C, and one 50 mg tablet of niacin (vitamin B₃). This niacin may be taken in addition to the normal 50 mg niacin tablets included in the patient's prescription. The pain triad may be taken up to five times per day, every four hours, if needed.

REFERENCES

1. M. Gerson, *A Cancer Therapy: Results of Fifty Cases and The Cure of Advanced Cancer by Diet Therapy: A Summary of Thirty Years of Clinical Experimentation*, 6th ed. (San Diego, CA: Gerson Institute, 1999), p. 209.
2. M. Gerson, *Gerson Therapy Handbook* (San Diego, CA: Gerson Institute, 1999), pp. 12-13.

CHAPTER 12

Why Does the Gerson Therapy Work?

The basic principles of the Gerson protocol are simple and clear and its practice has been yielding remarkable results for more than 80 years. However, the question remains: Is there any current scientific research to confirm the methods Dr. Gerson developed partly intuitively, partly through constant study and clinical observation, but without sophisticated research facilities, all those decades ago? Putting it simply, has anyone discovered just why this therapy works?

The answer is yes. Since Dr. Gerson's death in 1959, a series of eminent scientists and researchers have made discoveries that confirmed one or another of Dr. Gerson's insights and methods. The sum total of these piecemeal discoveries explains why his protocol, used in its entirety, is so effective. We now present a sample of the most striking scientific endorsements.

In the late '70s, the physicist, mathematician and biophysicist Freeman Widener Cope, MD, wrote in a paper stating that, **in cell damage of any kind, the same responses may occur in cells throughout the body: "First the cell will lose potassium, second the cell will accept sodium and third, the cell will swell with too much water (cellular** edema). **When the cell has swollen with too much water, energy production is inhibited, along with protein synthesis and lipid (fat) metabolism.** *Gerson was able to manipulate tissue damage syndrome, which he recognized clinically in the 1920s, by his dietary management, eliminating sodium, supplementing a high potassium diet with additional potassium amendments and finding a way to remove toxins from the body via the liver.*"[1] [Emphasis added.] This is a remarkably concise justification of all of Dr. Gerson's methods, including severe restriction of animal proteins, which the damaged cell cannot handle, the reason for increased potassium intake and the need for liver detoxification.

Important research justifying Dr. Gerson's withholding of animal protein was carried out by Robert A. Good, MD, of the University of Minnesota, who is known as "the father of modern immunology." He set up a guinea pig experiment, feeding one group of animals protein-free lab chow, while the other group received the normal variety of food. Dr. Good expected to failure of the animals' immune system on the protein-free regime, but the opposite happened. The guinea pigs' thymus lymphocytes became tremendously active and remained aggressively so for a long time. Dr. Good realized that he had stimulated immunity by the dietary restriction of animal protein, thus confirming the rightness of the Gerson protocol's identical insight.[2]

Gerson patients do receive adequate amounts of easily absorbed plant proteins contained in the fresh vegetable juices, potatoes and oatmeal that are essential parts of their diet. It is a widespread mistake to believe that only animal foods contain protein. On the contrary, food animals, such as cattle, pigs and sheep, are vegetarians!

One of the most important techniques of the Gerson Therapy is detoxification via the liver/bile through the use of coffee enemas. Dr. Gerson knew that these dilate the bile ducts, thus allowing the liver to release toxic accumulations. **His discovery was confirmed more recently by three scientists—Wattenberg, Sparmins and Lam3—from the Department of Pathology, University of Minnesota, who showed that rectal coffee administration stimulates an enzyme system (glutathione S-transferase) in the liver, which is able to remove toxic free radicals from the bloodstream.**

The normal activity of this enzyme is increased by 600% to 700% by the coffee enema, hence vastly increased detoxification results.

Coffee is also rich in potassium, which helps prevent intestinal cramping by boosting the potassium content of deficient smooth muscles in the colon.

REFERENCES

1. Freeman Widener Cope, "Pathology of structured water and associated cations in cells (the tissue damage syndrome) and its medical treatment," *Physiological Chemistry and Physics* 9 (6) (1977): 547-553.
2. Robert A. Good, MD, *The Influence of Nutrition on Development of Cancer Immunity and Resistance to Mesenchymal Diseases* (New York: Raben Press, 1982).
3. V. L. Sparmins, L. K. T. Lam and L. W. Wattenberg, "Proceedings of the American Association of Cancer Researchers and the American Society of Clinical Oncology," *Abstract* 22 (1981): 114, 453.

CHAPTER 13

Why the Gerson Therapy Is Salt-Free

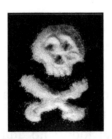

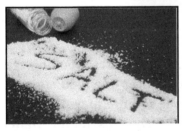

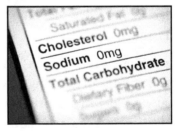

The Potassium/Sodium Metabolism

O ur entire metabolism depends on the constant exchange of nutrients and waste material between the trillions of cells of our entire organ system and the bloodstream. The blood carries nutrients and oxygen to each cell, and subsequently carries the waste products back out of the tissues for excretion, serving the entire body's needs. **This amazing exchange is highly dependent on the potassium/sodium ability to attract and move between the cells and the bloodstream.**

Blood—and the body's other essential fluid, serum—need to contain sodium minerals while, within every cell, potassium has to be available in abundance. The exchange between the body fluids and cells can only take place when the sodium in the liquid releases the nutrients (and picks up the waste products) because these two minerals produce the transport. For this reason, sodium must stay in the fluids and potassium in the tissues!

Natural nutrients, organic fruit and vegetables combine to produce the correct balance between these two essential minerals. Fluids make up about 10% of the body mass; the tissues about 90%.

If the human being eats correctly, a vegetarian, salt-free diet provides the optimum level of these minerals: about 10% of the diet is high in sodium (provided by natural foods; no addition is needed) while the remainder, about 90%, is high in potassium (provided by organic, unsalted fruit and vegetables).

The problem arises when artificial processes, cooking, canning, freezing, bottling, preserving, etc., take over our food supply. Potassium is always lost in the process, while sodium in constantly increasing quantities is regularly added. Clearly, this totally changes the body's normal chemistry and is the beginning of all disease.

Why a Salt-Free Diet?

Salt has been in use by humans for longer than recorded history, mostly as a flavor enhancer for food but for many other purposes as well, including food preservation, pest control, toothpaste, scouring powder and road and walkway ice melting. **The purpose we address here is its use—indeed overuse—in food preparation and preservation.**

Before refrigeration was invented and widely available, salt (sodium chloride) was one of the most popular means of food preservation, allowing meat, fish and other edible substances to be produced in one part of the world, then shipped to and consumed in another, or to be produced in time of plenty and preserved for use in a time of scarcity. In addition, salt has properties that suppress unpleasant tastes, so it makes some foods more palatable or even tasty. When it was widely used as a preservative, we became habituated to the "salty" taste, and food doesn't taste as "good" without added salt.

Over time, the human palate loses its sensitivity to salt, so the tendency is for the user to use more and more of the substance to maintain the "salty" flavor he seeks. However, there is a problem with the widespread and habitual use of salt. **It has been long recognized that there is a strong relationship between salt and high blood pressure.**[1] If you have high blood pressure, one of the first recommendations a physician will make is to lower your salt intake. In modern culture, this is no easy task.

Salt is composed of two elements, both very active chemically: sodium and chlorine (table salt is sodium chloride or NaCl; Na = sodium and Cl = chlorine). Each of these two elements is harmful to your body's metabolism in its own way.

Chlorine has the direct effect of driving essential iodine from the thyroid, dangerously reducing thyroid function. Sodium, meanwhile, is an enzyme inhibitor[2] with much more far-reaching effects. It promotes tissue damage syndrome by disrupting the metabolism, energy production, nutrition and waste flow of each and every cell in your body, promotes edema by retaining about 15 times its own weight in water and is essential for the growth of cancer cells.

Its opposite chemical element is potassium, which is necessary in large amounts for our health and well-being. In fact, some medical studies have disputed the need to reduce the amount of ingested salt, instead suggesting that what is important is the *balance* between salt and potassium intake.[3] The Standard American Diet (SAD) is very poor in potassium and very high in sodium, setting up a rich environment for development of chronic diseases.

Dr. Gerson saw the damage that high sodium did in a human body, as well as that done by a lack of potassium, and insisted that his patients avoid salt and all sodium compounds completely. He determined that the human body, which actually needs a certain amount of sodium to function properly, requires only about 200 mg (about 1/150 of an ounce) per day of sodium, an amount contained easily in green leafy vegetables.[4] The SAD, on the other hand, contains between 3,400 and 10,000 mg of sodium daily, an overdose of between 17 and 50 times![5] No matter what substance you ingest, even if it is good for you, an overdose of 50-fold will surely cause serious damage in the long term, and often in the short term as well.

The number of sodium compounds available to us in our foods, particularly processed and restaurant foods, is very high. Not only are we awash in table salt, we must add to that MSG, sodium saccharine, baking soda, and a host of food-processing chemicals containing sodium. Toothpaste contains sodium fluoride—a compound so much more toxic than table salt that it is often used as rat poison![6]

The result is that we cannot avoid this toxic substance without carefully selecting and eating fresh, organic food that we prepare ourselves. In fact, **the great majority of our sodium intake is from processed and restaurant foods.** The habitual use of the salt shaker present on almost every dining table in the country adds further to the toxic load.

Food processing, meantime, removes potassium from the foods and adds sodium compounds for such reasons as flavor enhancement, preservative or cosmetic functions and texture modification. This upends the potassium-sodium balance in the food we eat, and thus the balance in our bodies. **Because our bodies expect that there will be plenty of potassium available from our foods (as is the case in natural, fresh foods), the body makes no special effort to retain it. Likewise, since sodium is rarely found in nature more than a few miles from a seashore, the body strongly retains the sodium it gets in order to provide the necessary balance. When the potassium-sodium ratio in the food** is reversed, we are flooded with sodium (that is retained) and starved of potassium (that easily leaches out of the system), with disastrous results for our bodies.

Dixon and Webb, in their book *Enzymes*, called sodium an "enzyme inhibitor" (another word for "poison"), while its chemical opposite, potassium, is an enzyme enabler.[7] Every chemical activity in our bodies is regulated and mediated by enzymes, which act as "spark plugs" or catalysts that promote the activity. Inhibiting an enzyme naturally inhibits or deactivates the enzyme's ability to promote or enable the activity for which it is responsible.

When you consider the myriad activities that need to proceed properly in our complex bodies in order to maintain their normal functioning, the failure of even one of these activities can have serious, even fatal, consequences. Snake venom, for instance, can interfere with the enzyme that enables the blood to transport oxygen. Even in an atmosphere abundant with oxygen, your body dies from the lack of oxygen transported to the cells. Other poisons interfere with blood clotting, our autonomic breathing system, nerve impulse transmission . . . the list is endless. **Sodium interferes with many enzymes, inhibiting or stopping many vital functions.**

In an effort to repair the damage to body functions caused by the vast sodium-potassium imbalance, Dr. Gerson gave his patients potassium compound as a water-based solution in doses that might be considered "heroic" by other physicians. Wary of the fact that medical students are shown how direct application of potassium chloride solution will stop a frog's heart, Gerson explored over 300 combinations of potassium salts to find one that would be safe in all circumstances. This solution consists of **33.3 grams of each: potassium gluconate, potassium acetate and potassium phosphate (monobasic), dissolved in 1 liter (~1 quart) of distilled water, resulting in an 0.1 molar solution that is added to most of the juices in a day of therapy.** The frog's heart notwithstanding, no patient has ever been harmed by this combination or dosage, even when they accidentally overdose by 10 times or more!

As the potassium is returned to the system, it reclaims its rightful place in the cell. The sodium is forced out of the cell (where it does not belong) back into the bloodstream (where it does), excess amounts of sodium are excreted and balance is restored. **When the potassium-sodium balance is restored, cell metabolism is normalized, restarting energy production, nutrients and waste products migrate across the cell membranes in the right directions and healing begins. The process is amazingly fast.**

Freeman Cope, MD, writing in the peer-reviewed journal, *Physiological Chemistry and Physics,* said, "The high potassium, low sodium diet of the Gerson Therapy has been observed experimentally to cure many cases of advanced cancer in man, but the reason was not clear. Recent studies [this was in 1978] from the laboratory of Dr. F. G. Ling and associates indicate that high potassium, low sodium environments can partially return damaged cell proteins to their normal undamaged configuration. Therefore, **the damage in other tissues, indicated by toxins and breakdown products from the cancer, is probably partly repaired by the Gerson Therapy through this mechanism.**"[8]

Around every tumor or arthritic joint, in most chronic viral conditions such as genital herpes and other long-standing pathologies, the patients' tissues that have lost potassium gain sodium and swell with too much water. It has been established in modern medicine that this is a physiological fact.[9]

When he studied tuberculous infections, Dr. Gerson observed the same phenomenon and recorded it in his published works. Around every tubercular cavern and cavity, he saw a puffy, malfunctioning sphere of adjacent tissue damaged by toxins escaping from the tuberculosis organism. Partial metabolites in the disease lesions cause difficulties because they are waste material that promote destructive processes when left in place. Their presence upsets otherwise normal tissue so that it, in turn, becomes damaged.

Since an ounce of sodium retains a pound of water in the cells, manifesting as edema, or swelling, when the excess sodium is eliminated, the water it has bound into the cells is also released. Because of this process, the patient can easily lose 8-10 pounds (3.5 to 4.5 kg) of retained water per day, until the excess sodium and associated edema are gone.

When the potassium-sodium balance is restored (primarily through the mechanism of salt deprivation and potassium supplementation), blood pressure normalizes quite quickly, in the order of days rather than weeks. **The Gerson salt-free diet is credited with reversing a very large number of diseases that by allopathic methods are considered "chronic" or "incurable," partially due to the importance of restoring the potassium-sodium balance.**

REFERENCES

1. "The positive relation of sodium intake and blood pressure, first recognized a century ago, has been well established in ecological, epidemiological, and experimental human studies." "Salt, Blood Pressure, and Human Health," Michael H. Alderman, Hypertension, *Amer. Heart Ass. Journal* (http://hyper.ahajournals.org/content/36/5/890.full. Mar. 2000).

2. Malcolm Dixon and Edwin C. Webb, *Enzymes* (London, New York and Bombay: Longmans Green and Co., 1966). p. 422-3.

3. Q. Yang, T. Liu, E. V. Kuklina, W. D. Flanders, Y. Hong, C. Gillespie, M. H. Chang, M. Gwinn, N. Dowling, M. J. Khoury and F. B. Hu. "Sodium and potassium intake and mortality among US adults: prospective data from the Third National Health and Nutrition Examination Survey." *Arch Intern Med.* 171(13):1183-91, July 11, 2011.

4. Max Gerson, "Sodium and Potassium Content of Foods" (table), *A Cancer Therapy: Results of Fifty Cases and The Cure of Advanced Cancer by Diet Therapy: A Summary of Thirty Years of Clinical Experimentation,* 6th ed. (San Diego, CA: Gerson Institute, 2002). p. 225-9.

5. "With so much salt in our food, it's no wonder the average American gets 3,436 milligrams of sodium per day. That's more than double the American Heart Association's recommended limit of 1,500 milligrams." "Processed Foods: Where is all that salt coming from?" American Heart Association, High Blood Pressure web page. Jul. 17, 2013 (www.heart.org/HEARTORG/Conditions/HighBloodPressure/PreventionTreatmentofHighBloodPressure/Processed-Foods-Where-is-all-that-salt-coming-from_UCM_426950_Article.jsp).

6. Carolyn Evans-Dean, "Fluoride in Rat Poison," *eHow home.* "Since the 1800s, fluoride has been a key component in rat poison and insecticides. When mixed into grain or other food, rats will readily consume the poison and die. This method was deemed to be preferable to other poisonous compounds because it was less hazardous to the humans and livestock that

might accidentally ingest it." (www.ehow.com/about_6544969_fluoride-rat-poison.html).

7. Note 2 (Dixon and Webb), supra.

8. F. W. Cope, "Pathology of structured water and associated cations in cells (the tissue damage syndrome) and its medical treatment." *Physiological Chemistry and Physics,* 9(6):547-53, 1977.

9. Ibid.

CHAPTER 14

The Gerson Household

W hether a patient is able to spend some time at a Gerson facility or decides to embark on the therapy at home, the longest part of the healing process—up to two years or more with malignant disease but much less with other chronic conditions—will have to take place in his or her residence. **For the duration of the treatment, the home needs to be turned into a kind of private clinic where everything serves the goal of getting well and nothing is allowed to interfere with that process.**

How do we go about that? Quite simply, we bear in mind that the twin pillars of the Gerson program are nutrition and detoxification. Since the patient is both toxic and nutritionally deficient, as a first task the household has to be cleared of all toxic chemicals and damaging materials or appliances. These are present in vast arrays in most modern households. Chemical cleansers, gadgets and labor-saving devices emitting harmful radiation or so-called electrosmog are used daily and taken for granted. We only get rid of these substances and devices when their dire effects on the body are understood.

The first pillar of the therapy is to provide the patient with hypernutrition and a suitably equipped kitchen. The kitchen is the all-important center where all foods and juices are prepared daily in large amounts.

Let us start by listing the correct equipment for a smoothly running, efficient Gerson kitchen.

Refrigerator

One very large or two average size refrigerators will be needed to store the large quantities of organic produce required. A cool, preferably dark, well-ventilated pantry or laundry room is ideal for storing root vegetables, which don't need refrigeration.

Juice Machines

As freshly made organic juices are one of the most important healing components of the Gerson program, they must be of the best possible quality. It is therefore vital to choose the most efficient juicer—one that will stand up to constant use over two years or so.

There are plenty of models on the market. The simplest and cheapest is the centrifugal type, one of the first to become widely available. It is wasteful, produces deficient, enzyme-poor juice and CANNOT be used for healing.

Another type is the Champion juicer, which extracts more minerals as well as more fluid. However, it is not satisfactory in itself, since what it produces is not so much juice as a mushy layer of vegetables on top of a watery base. **Even so, the Champion juicer can be used, but only as a grinder.** The machine comes with a plate that can be placed under the base where the strainer is usually located, releasing the ground-up pulpy material.

This pulp has to be put through a hand-operated press, based on a hydraulic jack, to squeeze the juice from the pulped vegetables.

The cost of the two items runs at about $600. The Champion juicer is widely available in the United States and in several other countries. For the manual press, contact The Juice Press Factory (www.juicepressfactory.com).

Other machines, imported from Korea and made in the United States, use two interlocking helical blades which grind against each other. They do a better extracting job than the Champion alone and may be used, especially if the patient is not suffering from cancer. However, these "one-process" juicers do not actually conform to Dr. Gerson's instruction to use a two-process method, consisting of a grinder and a press, for obtaining the best juice. These juicers claim to extract more enzymes than the Norwalk (below), but no mention is made of the equally important mineral extraction. The cost of these machines is between $750 and $900.

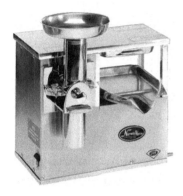

The best two-process juicer is the Norwalk Hydraulic Press Juicer, which is also most attractively styled with a stainless steel exterior or a wood grain plastic outer cover. Naturally, in either model, all parts of the machine that come in contact with food are made from stainless steel. The Norwalk is fully automatic, with a simple lever activating the press. Well serviced and guaranteed, it is also the most expensive juicer ($2,395 to $2,495). The stainless steel exterior model also has a lever that adjusts it to the 220 to 240 volt current used in Europe. For information, call (800) 405-8423 (outside the United States, call +1 (760) 436-9683) or visit the Norwalk Juicers California Web site (www.nwjcal.com).

For patients on a tight budget, used Norwalk Juicers are sometimes available directly from Norwalk (www.norwalkjuicers.com/used-juicers) or possibly from reseller on eBay (www.eBay.com) or Craigslist (www.craigslist.com).

Taking Care of Your Juice Machine

Aside from your normal routine of maintaining maximum cleanliness in the kitchen, **it is especially important to keep your juicer clean and** free from dried-up juice and/or fibers. Since these are raw, they can easily spoil, dry and attract flies and other insects and germs.

To avoid contamination, the juicer must be cleaned after each use. This should not take up much extra time since those parts of the machine that come in contact with fruits and vegetables are made of stainless steel and are easy to take apart, rinse, dry and reassemble for the next juice.

Use only clean sponges or cloths and reserve them for the juicer alone. **Do not use soap or detergent for each cleansing because it is highly important that not even the smallest amount of soap or cleanser remains on the parts that come in contact with the vegetables.** If you use a Norwalk juicer, remember to wipe the press plate at the top.

The juice cloths should be rinsed carefully in clean—not soapy—water after each pressing and kept in the freezer until the next juicing. It is best to have separate cloths for the apple/carrot or plain carrot juice and for the green juice.

At night, after all the juices have been made, you may use slightly soapy water for the day's final cleansing; afterwards, rinse thoroughly to make sure that no soapy film remains. Even a small residue of soap getting into the juices could cause the patient diarrhea, cramps or worse. The same applies to the juice cloths. Wash them in slightly soapy water and rinse carefully to get rid of any soapy residue. Keep the cloths in the freezer overnight.

If you use a grinder (i.e., a Champion) and a press operated by a hydraulic system, the same rules apply. Keep both machines scrupulously clean and clear of soap.

Stove and Oven: Electric or Gas?

Neither type is ideal. The cooking temperature is easier to control with a gas stove. However, gas burns oxygen, and if the patient spends time in the kitchen, the oxygen-depleted air is likely to prove harmful. The kitchen has to be well ventilated, which may be difficult on cold, winter days. **The installation of a room ozone generator in the kitchen/living area is recommended in order to restore a better oxygen level.**

Caution: If the ozone level is too high, it could be set on fire by open flames.

Electric stoves or ovens are more expensive than gas to operate in most areas of the United States. Their advantage is that they are cleaner and don't use up oxygen. However, the cooking temperature, so very important for the correct preparation of vegetables, is more difficult to control on electric stoves.

Microwave Oven

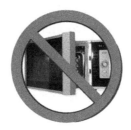

Because of its speed and apparent efficiency, this gadget has spread to countless kitchens in the United States and elsewhere, without knowing its serious health hazards. Since many microwave ovens carry an "Underwriters Laboratories" guarantee of safety, the general public is led to believe that these ovens are safe to use. This is not the case.

Research carried out in Switzerland[1] and elsewhere has shown that microwaves cause harmful chemical reactions in food, damaging nutrients, producing unnatural molecules and making natural amino acids toxic. The heat is uneven; it doesn't reach the middle of solid food but instead produces "hot spots." Liquids can overheat and cause severe burns when the food is removed. To make things worse, these ovens emit radiation into the kitchen area even when not in use and "cook the cook."[2] **(It is an interesting fact that, for health reasons, microwave ovens were banned in the former Soviet Union as far back as 1976!)**[3]

If you own one, get rid of it. If it is not removable, unplug it and don't be tempted to use it under any circumstances.

Pots and Utensils

Any contact of food with aluminum causes small amounts (or with some vegetables, such as tomatoes, large amounts) of aluminum to be dissolved and released into the food. This metal is highly toxic; it causes brain damage and is believed to play a role in causing Alzheimer's.[4]

Discard any and all aluminum items and don't allow aluminum foil to come into contact with food. Use stainless steel pots, preferably with heavy "waterless" bottoms, or glass (Pyrex) or enameled cast iron pots. Stainless steel cooking utensils or wooden spoons are best. Use silver flatware, if available (small amounts of colloidal silver, released from silver forks, spoons and knives are valuable stimulants for the immune system).

Do not use pressure cookers; they work at a very high temperature, which damages nutrients. One of the basic Gerson rules is to cook food very slowly, at a low temperature, to avoid such damage. The glaze used on some crockpots is toxic[5]—best to steer clear of them.

Distillers

Surprising though this may sound, Gerson patients don't drink water. There are two reasons for this. On the one hand, their daily intake of many glasses of freshly made organic juices and fluid-rich soup, salads and fruit provide them with all the top-quality nutritious liquid they need. **On the other hand, water would only dilute their already deficient digestive juices without supplying any nutrients.** However, water is used in the Gerson Therapy in cooking—to make soups, teas and, of course, enemas—and it is vitally important to ensure the purity of this water.

There are various filter systems on the market, including reverse osmosis, which can only be used if the local water supply is guaranteed free from highly harmful fluoride. **The safest way to ensure freedom from impurities, toxic chemicals and, above all, fluoride is to set up a home distiller.**

Many kinds of distillers are available in various price ranges. Choice must depend on cost and on the amount of water the household may need. The patient alone will use 2 to 3 gallons in every 24-hour period, and more if other family members also eat Gerson food and/or wish to use enemas.

A distiller needs an electric connection and an extra water faucet, and many patients install theirs in the laundry room or garage. **The machine needs to be detached and cleaned every three days.** Seeing the sludge left behind will convince anyone of the need to purify water as thoroughly as possible.

Distillation works by heating water to the point of becoming steam, which is run through a tube that causes it to cool and condense back into water. Since minerals, various impurities and additives do not turn into steam, they stay behind, leaving the cooled, condensed steam free from harmful components. However, volatile liquids, such as benzene fractions, also boil away and are condensed back into the purified water.

To remove such items, make sure the distiller you choose contains a carbon filtration system, so that when the condensed water drips back into a fresh container, it passes through the carbon filter, which removes the unwanted volatile items.

It is sometimes claimed by health professionals that distilled water "removes minerals from the body" and shouldn't be used,[6] but they are wrong. The minerals found in water (e.g., sodium or calcium) are generally inorganic and are therefore poorly absorbed or downright harmful. On the other hand, the patient is virtually flooded with the easily absorbed organic minerals contained in the large amount of juices drunk throughout the day; the "loss" of minerals contained in tap water is actually a gain.

Cleaning Chemicals

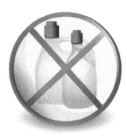

Cleanliness is of course all important in the Gerson household but, as stated before, **special care must be taken not to use toxic products. Here are the ones to avoid:**

Chlorine

Chlorine is not only bleach but also a powerful disinfectant, able to kill or control all kinds of germs. For that reason, it is present in almost all kitchen cleansers (and in swimming pools and tap water!). **Chlorine is harsh and unsafe, able to displace iodine from the thyroid gland and must be avoided.** There are a few kitchen cleansers that do not contain chlorine, so try to find one. You can also produce your own by mixing half malt vinegar with half water and decanting it into a spray-pump bottle to clean glass or polish kitchen surfaces, but keep it off wood. Plain soap and hot water are also recommended.

To remove lime scale, soak a piece of cotton in white vinegar, wrap it around the faucets in your kitchen or bathroom and leave it for 30 minutes. Wash it off with soap and water.

Clean stainless steel pans with olive oil. The result is stunning, but use the oil sparingly and be careful to clean it all off.

Solvents

Paint solvents, grease or glue solvents are all toxic and damaging to the patient. If one has to be used, take it outside and don't allow it to evaporate in the kitchen.

Dishwasher Soap

Most dishwashers are equipped with two wash cycles followed by one rinse cycle. Since the Gerson Therapy does not involve the use of greasy food or baking dishes, **it is best to use one wash cycle and ensure that the soap is cleared by using two rinse cycles.** In that way, the dishwasher soap should be completely eliminated, with no toxic residue remaining on dishes.

Laundry Soap and Bleach

If the laundry is washed in a washing machine, the same applies to dishwasher soap. You can use any appropriate soap and even add bleach, if needed, as long as it is inside the machine and the patient doesn't smell it. **(If the patient can smell it, he or she is getting some into their system.)** Make very sure that the laundry is thoroughly rinsed, possibly running a second rinse cycle.

Fabric Softeners

These should be avoided, whether in liquid form or as drying sheets. Either way, they leave a chemical film, which never washes out completely. They are also irritating to sensitive individuals (e.g., asthma sufferers). As a harmless alternative, add 1/4 cup of distilled white vinegar to the wash cycle. This softens your clothes and also gets rid of static cling. If you are washing delicate items (e.g., those marked "hand wash"), use a mild soap and wear rubber gloves.

Dry Cleaning

As this is done outside the home, it doesn't directly affect the patient. However, when dry-cleaned items are brought home, it is wise to leave them outdoors without their plastic covers to let them air out and get rid of any remaining chemicals.

Aerosols and Sprays

Do not use any of these. Once the spray is distributed in the air, it is impossible to avoid inhaling it. Obviously, the toxic pesticide sprays are the most dangerous. However, any cleaning chemicals (e.g., window cleaners and oven cleaners) that are sprayed will go into the air and be inhaled.

If a window cleaner is used, pour a little on a cloth and wipe the window clean without spraying. As a suggestion, windows can be cleaned and completely streak free by pouring white vinegar on some slightly crumpled newspaper and wiping the window (with light pressure) until clean.

Oven cleaning is not much of a problem, since the Gerson food is clear of fats and doesn't cause deposits on the oven walls.

The Bathroom

Chlorine-containing cleansers should not be used in the bathroom. Disinfect with 3% commercial hydrogen peroxide.

It is important to note that your skin is a semipermeable membrane, which means that everything you put on your skin is absorbed into your body. This includes all of the chemicals contained in your soaps, shampoos, toothpaste, creams, balms, cosmetics, fragrances, aftershaves, colognes, convenience wipes and more. **As much as possible, patients on the Gerson Therapy should only use organic soaps and shampoos with a minimum amount of chemicals and fragrances.** Gerson patients should make sure to avoid all spray deodorizers, antiperspirants and underarm deodorants.

Men should use old-style spreadable shaving soaps, not products that come in aerosol cans or sprays. Avoid aerosol aftershaves and perfumes and any scented lotions. Only use plain, white, unscented toilet paper.

There are numerous organic soaps and shampoos available today, and your local organic food store should have a full range for you to pick from. Also, a quick search on the Internet will provide an abundance of chemical-free items that will suit your personal preferences.

Dental Care

Brushing and Flossing

Good dental hygiene is important on the Gerson Therapy. **Patients should take care to brush and floss regularly** as bacteria may form in between teeth and gums and may enter the bloodstream. Patients are also advised to rinse with distilled water and dry brush after each juice to prevent cavities that may arise from natural sugar in the carrots and apples that accumulates on the teeth and around the gums.

Fluoride Toothpaste

Patients must not use fluoride toothpaste. The fluoride in toothpaste is as toxic as the fluoride in water, and will be absorbed by the mucous membranes in the mouth. To illustrate this point, the packaging of toothpaste containing fluoride displays a warning that if you eat or swallow more than a pea-sized dollop of toothpaste, you should call your local poison control center immediately.

> # WARNING
> **Keep out of the reach of Children under 6 years of age.**
> **If you accidentaly swallow more than is used for**
> **brushing, get medical help or contact a poison**
> **control center right away.**
> **When using this product, if irritation occurs**
> **discontinue use.**

Mercury Amalgam Fillings

Warning regarding the removal of mercury amalgam fillings: Gerson patients must not have their silver amalgam fillings removed until they have been on the therapy at least nine to 12 months. Even with the best precautions, the high-speed drills used during the removal process will:

- Release poisonous mercury gas that will be inhaled by the patient

- Create microparticles of mercury amalgam that may be absorbed in the mouth, inhaled and/or swallowed

- Create medium-sized particles of mercury amalgam that can be swallowed

Mercury is a poisonous neurotoxin, and even small amounts ingested during the removal of fillings can make normal healthy individuals very sick. With Gerson patients, it can have serious consequences.

Polishing Fillings During Dental Cleanings

Patients should never allow their "silver" amalgam fillings to be polished, cleaned or abraded for any reason. This will remove the body's natural covering material and the slight surface oxidation that helps to keep some the mercury from leaching into the body.

Baking Soda

A question we receive quite often is whether patients can use baking soda in place of toothpaste. The answer is NO! What is baking soda? Sodium bicarbonate—a sodium-based compound—must be avoided as it will be absorbed in the mouth, sabotaging the healing process.

Living Area

Many kinds of toxic damage can be caused inadvertently in the living room. **One possible culprit is furniture polish, which contains solvent and must be banished.** Carpet cleaning presents another potential hazard. Do not use (or allow cleaning services to use) chemical cleaners, only soapy solutions.

Very serious toxic damage has been caused by new carpeting,[7] most of which is impregnated with toxic pesticides or other chemicals to resist staining. If it is absolutely necessary to install new carpeting, track down nontoxic kinds. Several manufacturers have been sued[8] for their carpets causing allergic reactions in sensitive people and, as a result, nontoxic carpets are now being produced.

An even more dangerous process is termite extermination. Some exterminators use a whole house cover and spread gas throughout the building. When the covers are removed, fresh air is allowed back in, but a lot of poison is left behind in upholstered furniture, carpets and drapes. It takes some six months or so to outgas! There are other nontoxic methods available (e.g., find out about the freezing approach).

Living room areas are often routinely treated to "air fresheners" via sprays or a chemical solid. Do not use either.

Whole House Painting

No part of the inside of the house should be painted while the patient is recovering. Walls may be washed down with mild soap; stains can be removed with a nontoxic cleanser. The house may not look perfect but, for the time being, the patient's recovery must be given absolute priority.

Outdoor Garden Sprays/Agricultural Pesticides

Some areas of daily life are beyond the caregiver's control, such as neighbors who spray their gardens with pesticides. If and when this happens, make sure that all windows are closed, and use the room air cleaner and ozone generator to protect the patient. A similar problem is caused by pesticide spraying of agricultural areas in the vicinity. In one such case, the recovering patient had a serious reaction and suffered a recurrence until she moved away (to live with her sister) for the time being, where she recovered again.

REFERENCES

1. Hans Hertel and Bernard H. Blanc, "Microwave Ovens" (Vol. 22, No. 2) and "Microwaves the Best Article Yet," Price-Pottenger Nutrition Foundation, *PPNF Journal* 24 (2) (Summer 2000).
2. Ibid.
3. Ibid.
4. Virginie Rondeau, Daniel Commenges, Hélène Jacqmin-Gadda and Jean-François Dartigues, "Relation between Aluminum Concentrations in Drinking Water and Alzheimer's Disease: An 8-year Follow-up Study," *American Journal of Epidemiology* 152 (2000): 59-66.
5. Dixie Farley, "Dangers of Lead Still Linger," U.S. Food and Drug Administration, *FDA Consumer* (January-February 1998) (www.cfsan.fda.gov/~dms/fdalead.html).
6. P. Airola, *How To Get Well* (Phoenix: Health Plus Publishers, 1974).
7. Cindy Duehring, "Carpet Concerns, Part Four: Physicians Speak Up As Medical Evidence Mounts," Environmental Access Research Network (Minot, ND) (www.holisticmed.com/carpet/tc4.txt).
8. Fluoride Action Network, Pesticide Project, Class Action Suit-PFOA (www.fluoridealert.org/pesticides/effect.pfos.classaction.htm).

CHAPTER 15

Forbidden Foods

A McDonald's "Breakfast for Under a Dollar"
actually costs much more than that. You have to
factor in the cost of coronary bypass surgery.

—*George Carlin*

Just as some foods, brilliantly combined in the Gerson protocol, are great healers, others are strictly excluded from the patient's diet. In his classic book, *A Cancer Therapy—Results of Fifty Cases,*[1] Dr. Gerson gives a long list of "Forbidden Foods." Actually, "Forbidden Items" would be a more accurate title, since the list is not limited to foodstuffs only. Newcomers to the Gerson program are understandably puzzled by some of these prohibitions, banning foods that are routinely eaten and even considered wholesome by the average "normal" citizen, so let's see why they must be excluded. Rules and regulations are easier to follow if we know the reasons behind them.

In fact, today's list of banned substances is longer than Dr. Gerson's original one. Since he wrote his book half a century ago, many changes have occurred that make healthy living increasingly difficult. The huge development of the food industry—with its vast range of additives, freely used in the ever-wider assortment of convenience foods—has changed people's eating habits for the worse, exposing consumers to the ill effects of what are politely called food cosmetics.

One of the worst—the highly toxic[2] sugar substitute aspartame, sold as NutraSweet, Spoonful, Equal—is contained in some 6,000[3] processed foods found on grocery shelves. Last, but far from least, all processed foods contain salt, the very substance that causes tissue damage syndrome and stimulates tumor growth.[4]

Added to this, the products of industrial agriculture carry heavy residues of toxic pesticides, herbicides, fungicides, growth promoters, hormones, antibiotics and any one of the thousands of substances allowed to be used by the Food and Drug Administration,[5] which are supposed to be harmless. **Indeed, some of these substances tested singly may prove to be harmless but, in combination with others, which is how people consume them in the real world, they add up to a poisonous cocktail.** Let's remember that all these chemicals are toxic and damaging to the liver, the very organ which the Gerson Therapy endeavors to heal and restore.

These are the two basic rules for Gerson patients:

1. All processed foods, whether they are canned, jarred, bottled, frozen, salted, refined, sulphured, smoked, pickled, irradiated, microwaved or otherwise treated, must be strictly avoided.

2. Only fruits and vegetables certified as organic must be used, for they are free of agricultural poisons and are grown in healthy soil, which contains all the necessary vitamins, enzymes, minerals, trace elements and microorganisms that are needed for optimum health.

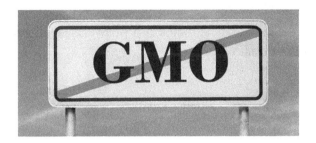

Admittedly, these days even organically cultivated soil does not contain the same level of useful minerals as it did even 15 years ago, but the great amount of organic food and juices that a Gerson patient is given daily makes up for the deficiencies.

As for the forbidden items, the harmful effects of tobacco and alcohol are too well known to need explanation. Next, sodium (salt) and fats of all kinds, except flaxseed oil, must be avoided. This, of course, brings into the group of forbidden foods many items that contain one or both of these two banned substances (e.g., avocados are rich in natural oil, which is fat). If you bear in mind the ban on fats and salt, the following list will make sense without detailed explanations.

To simplify matters even further, let's repeat loud and clear: Only foods that contribute to health and healing are allowed; all else is banned.

Forbidden Foods and Nonfood Items

- All processed foods (premade, heat and eat, ready to eat and prepackaged industrial foods)
- Alcohol
- Avocados
- Berries (except currants)
- Bicarbonate of soda (baking soda) in foods, toothpaste and gargle

- Bottled and canned commercial beverages (soft drinks)
- Cake, candy, chocolate and all kinds of sweets (high sugar and fats; no nutritional value)
- Cheese
- Cocoa
- Coffee for drinking
- Cosmetics, hair dyes and permanents
- Cream
- Cucumber (poorly digested)
- Dried fruit (if sulphured or glazed with oil)
- Drinking water (see the section on distillers in Chapter 14, "The Gerson Household," p. 123)
- Epsom salts (also for foot baths)
- Fats and oils (sole exception: flaxseed oil, as prescribed)
- Flour (white and wholemeal; also flour products such as pasta)
- Fluoride, in water and toothpaste
- Herbs (except permitted ones) (see Chapter 17, "Preparing Food and Juices —The Basic Rules," p. 147)
- Ice cream and sherbet (artificial flavors, sweeteners and cream)
- Legumes (only occasional use in latter part of therapy)
- Milk (also defatted or low fat)
- Mushrooms (fungi, not vegetables)
- Nuts (high in fats; wrong configuration of proteins)
- Orange and lemon rind (contains aromatic oils)
- Pickles
- Pineapples (high in aromatics)
- Salt and all salt substitutes

- Soy and all soy products (e.g., tofu, soy milk and flour)

- Most spices (high in aromatics)

- Sugar (refined white)

- Tea (black and green if caffeinated; black tea is high in natural fluoride)

- Wheatgrass juice

Dr. Gerson's total ban on soy and all soy products may sound surprising at first, since soy has the much-publicized reputation of being an ideal vegetarian food (i.e., high in protein and low in fat and cholesterol). It is also consumed in the Far East where cancer incidence is considerably lower than in the West.

However, the truth behind this commercially motivated publicity is very different (soy is very big business in the United States, where 60% of supermarket foods contain some form of it). In fact, soy is high in oil and contains at least 30 allergy-causing proteins, which can cause severe damage[6] to susceptible individuals. Soy also contains phytic acid, which blocks the uptake of important minerals; enzyme inhibitors, which annul the healing power of the vital oxidizing enzymes contained in the juices; and a clot-promoting substance, which causes red blood cells to clump together—ample justification for the total exclusion of soy from the Gerson protocol.

Please note: **Two "home-grown" foods—sprouted seeds and wheatgrass juice—which became fashionable some 20 years ago and are considered wholesome and nutritious, must not be used by Gerson patients.** Our experience has shown that, unfortunately, both have harmful side effects.

Sprouts were eaten in large amounts by two Gerson patients at our hospital instead of the usual salads at lunch and dinner. Within a short time, both developed recurrences of their primary diseases (i.e., lupus and cervical cancer) after being symptom-free for months. Other lupus patients, getting sprouts from the hospital kitchen in their salads and juices, stopped responding to the treatment and even got worse.

Shortly afterwards, researchers[7] discovered that sprouts contain immature proteins, called L-canavanine, which suppress the immune system. At the Gerson hospital, sprouts were immediately banned and the earlier problems disappeared at once. All past patients were also advised to stop using sprouts in their diet.

Wheatgrass juice contains many valuable nutrients, but it is difficult to digest, tends to irritate the stomach and can only be taken in 1-ounce portions. Used as a rectal implant, it can cause serious irritation. Besides, the Gerson green juice (consisting of salad greens, chard, a little green pepper, some red cabbage and an apple per 8-ounce glass) (see Chapter 17, "Preparing Food and Juices —The Basic Rules," p. 147) is highly digestible, contains similar nutrients and can be enjoyed in four 8-ounce portions a day without unpleasant side effects—excellent reasons for not using wheatgrass juice.

Temporarily Forbidden Foods While on Gerson Healing Program

- Butter
- Cottage cheese (salt-free, defatted)
- Eggs
- Fish
- Meat
- Yogurt (and other fermented milk products)

Forbidden Personal and Household Items

- Aerosols of all types
- Carpeting (new)
- Chemical cleansers (see Chapter 14, "The Gerson Household," p. 123)
- Chlorine bleach

- Cosmetics

- Ointments

- Paint (fresh)

- Perfumes

- Pesticide sprays

- Wood preservatives

REFERENCES

1. M. Gerson, *A Cancer Therapy: Results of Fifty Cases and The Cure of Advanced Cancer by Diet Therapy: A Summary of Thirty Years of Clinical Experimentation,* 6th ed. (San Diego, CA: Gerson Institute, 1999).

2. Aspartame (NutraSweet) Toxicity Info Center (www.holisticmed.com/ aspartame); *see also* H. J. Roberts, MD, "Does Aspartame Cause Human Brain Cancer?," *Journal of Advancement in Medicine* 4 (4) (Winter 1991).

3. Joseph Mercola, MD, "Can Rumsfeld 'Defend' Himself Against Aspartame Lawsuit?" (www.mercola.com/2005/jan/12/rumsfeld_aspartame.htm); *see also* Note 2 (Roberts), supra.

4. Freeman Widener Cope, "A medical application of the Ling Association-Induction Hypothesis: the high potassium, low sodium diet of the Gerson cancer therapy," *Physiological Chemistry and Physics* 10 (5) (1978): 465-468.

5. Healthy Eating Adviser: Food Additives (www.healthyeatingadvisor.com/ food-additives.html) (updated 2006).

6. "Soy Dangers Summarised," SoyOnlineService (www.soyonlineservice.co.nz/03summary.htm).

7. M. R. Malinow, E. J. Bardana, Jr., B. Pirofsky, S. Craig and P. McLaughlin, "Systemic lupus erythematosus-like syndrome in monkeys fed alfalfa sprouts: role of a nonprotein amino acid," *Science* 216 (4544) (Apr. 23, 1982): 415-417.

CHAPTER 16

Happy Foods

Even the highest medicine can cure only eight
or nine out of 10 sicknesses. The sicknesses that
medicine cannot cure can be cured only by foods.

—The Yellow Emperor's Classic of Internal
Medicine *(Chinese, circa 400 B.C.)*

Food is Better Medicine than Drugs

—*Title of book by leading British
nutritionist Patrick Holford*

"So what *is* there to eat?" asks the startled newcomer to the Gerson way of life, after reading the list of forbidden foods in the preceding chapter. That is an important question to ponder. It shows how alienated one can become from a natural way of eating and, above all, from the huge range of available plant foods, rightly called the vegetable kingdom (which, in this instance, also includes fruits). It is a fair guess that the majority of people in the so-called developed world regard vegetables as no more than incidentals that accompany a main course of fish or meat, while fruits are only considered if there is no dessert offered. This is the moment to think again—and to make some delightful discoveries.

The fact is that plant foods, which are the basis of the Gerson regime, are superior to animal-based ones. Besides being lighter, more pure and easier to digest and absorb, each one contains a subtle mixture of vitamins, enzymes, minerals and trace elements, which work in synergy (i.e., in cooperation) and supply the depleted organism with valuable nutrients. Only when the nonhealing—in fact, harmful—food items are excluded, the wide range and variety of plant foods become clear. It is their usefulness as well as their beauty that need to be acknowledged.

Try to look at a display of fresh, organic fruits and vegetables with the eyes of an artist. Note the glowing colors and varied shapes of golden carrots, deep red cabbages, creamy cauliflowers with their light green collars, beige pears, multicolored apples and translucent green grapes—the range is vast, and eye appeal adds a great deal to the enjoyment of the produce.

There is another happy surprise that awaits the novice explorer of the vegetable kingdom: the discovery of the true flavor of vegetables and fruits. At first, without salt and pepper, plant foods taste bland—and, frankly, boring—but they are neither. However, a lifetime of excessive use of salt deadens the taste buds of the tongue until they are unable to convey the true taste of any food, and even the salt intake has to be continually increased to have any effect. On the salt-free Gerson regime, it takes a week or so for the paralyzed taste buds to recover. Once that happens, fruits and vegetables suddenly begin to taste more interesting. At the same time, one's sense of smell also becomes more acute and contributes to the enjoyment of every meal.

"Let your food be your medicine, and let your medicine be your food," said Hippocrates, the father of modern medicine, some 2,500 years ago. [Emphasis added.] We might add, "Let your medicine consist of happy foods only!"

CHAPTER 17

Preparing Food and Juices –The Basic Rules

A first-rate soup is more
creative than a second-rate painting.

—Abraham Maslow

A ssuming that your kitchen is now fully equipped for your healing Gerson routine, and that you have banished from your home all forbidden foods and substances, the moment has come to find out about the all-important task of food preparation. The rules are simple, but they must be observed faithfully to secure the best results.

All food must be organic and as fresh as possible. Ideally, we should be able to gather fresh, living food from our own organic gardens; unfortunately, this is not an ideal world and we must compromise. The next best thing is to shop frequently for salad and leaf vegetables in smallish amounts so there is no need to keep them for any length of time. Apples, pears, oranges and root vegetables can be stored for a while without significant loss of quality.

The two most important basic rules of food preparation are the following:

1. All foods must be prepared with great care in order to preserve nutrients as much as possible. **Cooking must be slow, using low heat**; *high temperatures alter nutrients in vegetables and cause them to be less easily absorbed.* Vegetables should not be peeled—valuable nutrients are contained in or immediately underneath their skins—and only washed or well scrubbed. Except for potatoes, corn and whole beets, which have to be boiled in sufficient water, vegetables are cooked with the minimum of water or soup stock (see "Special Soup or Hippocrates Soup," p. 152) or on a bed of sliced onions and tomatoes, which release enough moisture to keep the vegetables from burning. **Remember that oxidation, with loss of nutrients, sets in as soon as you cut into a vegetable or fruit; only start chopping when you are ready to cook.**

2. Food must be tasty, varied and enjoyable to make up for being very different from the so-called normal Western diet. Variety helps to stimulate appetite. It also supplies a wide range of minerals and trace elements needed by the body to heal. Remember the importance of eye appeal! Salads in particular can be made truly tempting by mixing green leaves with chopped tomatoes and multicolored peppers, adding radishes and a smattering of chives. (For further ideas, see Chapter 28, "Recipes," p. 209.)

A small vase of flowers on the dining table can work wonders in making the meal taste even better.

The Gerson diet strikes a fine balance between raw and cooked foods. The ample main meals may suggest to some patients that much of their food is cooked, but this is not the case. Meals begin with huge helpings of raw salad and end with raw fruit, and the daily ration of 13 glasses of freshly made juice is as raw as can be. **Cooked foods are necessary. Dr. Gerson's experience showed that patients do not digest well if given only raw foods along with the juices.** In fact, cooked foods provide additional variety and enable patients to eat more than they would on an exclusively raw diet. They also supply soft bulk, which promotes the digestion of the raw foods and juices.

The most popular item on the list of cooked foods is the "Special Soup or Hippocrates Soup" (p. 152) that helps to detoxify the kidneys and is highly comforting, especially in cold weather. All cooked foods serve as a kind of "blotting paper" in the stomach, helping to deal with the constant intake of large amounts of juice. Even so, cooked foods only account for some 3 to 4 pounds of the patient's daily consumption, while raw foods, mostly made into juices, represent some 17 pounds!

The All-Important Juices

Only four kinds of juice are used in the treatment of all categories of patients, except for a few minor exceptions. The basic juices are:

- **Apple/carrot juice**
- **Carrot-only juice**
- **Green juice**
- **Orange juice**

Occasionally, for special cases, a different juice may have to be substituted. For example, diabetics receive grapefruit juice instead of orange juice, since grapefruit contains less sugar; sometimes a fruit juice, such as apple juice, is given to patients with collagen diseases who should not drink citrus juice.

Apple/Carrot Juice

Use approximately 8 ounces each of carrots and apples. Wash and brush (do not peel), grind to a pulp and place in a cloth supplied with the press-type juicer to press. Serve and drink immediately.

Carrot-Only Juice

Use approximately 10-12 ounces of carrots. Wash and brush (do not peel), grind to a pulp and place in a cloth supplied with the press-type juicer to press. Serve and drink immediately.

Green Juice

Use romaine, red leaf lettuce, endive, escarole, two to three leaves of red cabbage, young inner beet tops, Swiss chard, a quarter of a small green pepper and watercress. Add one medium apple when grinding. Procure as many of these materials as possible. If some of the above items are not available, do not use substitutes, such as spinach or celery. Grind the material to a pulp and place in a cloth for pressing. This juice must be drunk immediately since its enzymes die quickly.

Orange (or Grapefruit) Juice

Use only a reamer-type juicer, electric or hand operated. **Do not squeeze the peel of the fruit. The aromatic oils contained in the skin are harmful and would interfere with the treatment.**

The Daily Routine

The typical average daily menu of the Gerson patient is as follows:

Breakfast

- A large bowl of oatmeal cooked in distilled water and sweetened with a little honey or dried fruit, presoaked (soak overnight in cold water, or pour boiling water over them)
- An 8-ounce glass of freshly squeezed orange juice
- Some additional raw or stewed fruit
- *Optional:* a slice of toasted, unsalted, organic rye bread

Lunch

- A large plate of mixed raw salad with flaxseed oil dressing (see the Flaxseed Oil and Lemon Juice Dressing recipe in Chapter 28, "Recipes," p. 219)

- 8 to 10 ounces of the "Special Soup or Hippocrates Soup" (see p. 152)

- Baked, boiled, mashed or otherwise prepared potato

- 1 to 2 freshly cooked vegetables

- Raw or stewed fruit for dessert

Dinner

- Follows the same order as lunch, but is varied with different vegetables and fruit for dessert

Please note: Either at lunch or dinner, and after the patient has consumed the necessary foods, *he or she may eat a second slice of unsalted, organic rye bread. However, bread should not satisfy the appetite or take the place of essential foods.*

Basic Recipes to Start You Off

For a full range of Gerson recipes, please see Chapter 28, "Recipes," p. 209. The following instructions are only meant to introduce the most fundamental items of the patient's essential daily menu.

Breakfast

For one person, put 5 ounces of rolled oats into 12 ounces of **distilled water**. Start with cold water, bring to a boil and let simmer for 6 to 8 minutes, stirring occasionally. Meanwhile, squeeze orange juice and add any prescribed medication(s) (see Chapter 19, "Medications," p. 165). Serve the oatmeal with presoaked (soak overnight in cold water, or pour boiling water over them and leave for a couple of hours until plump), unsulphured dried fruit (e.g., apricots, apple rings, prunes, raisins and mango), or use raw or stewed apple or stewed plums, or fresh fruit in season (e.g., peaches, nectarines, grapes or pears) **Do not use berries.** Up to 2 teaspoons a day of permitted sweeteners (e.g., honey, maple syrup, spray-dried cane juices sold as sucanat (an organic dried cane sugar) and rapadura, or unsulphured molasses) may be used.

Lunch

For the salad, cut up, slice and mix varied lettuces, such as red leaf lettuce, Romaine, escarole, salad bowl and endive. Add to the mixture chopped green onions, radishes, a little celery, some tomatoes, cauliflower florets, slices of green pepper and watercress. For the dressing (see the Flaxseed Oil and Lemon Juice Dressing recipe in Chapter 28, "Recipes," p. 219), mix 1 tablespoon of flaxseed oil (during the first month of the therapy; afterwards, reduce to 2 teaspoons) with apple cider or red wine vinegar, or lemon or lime juice. Add garlic to taste.

"Special Soup or Hippocrates Soup" (below) is to be eaten twice daily throughout the treatment. To save time and effort, prepare enough for two days (i.e., four portions). It will keep in the refrigerator overnight for the next day.

Special Soup or Hippocrates Soup

1 medium celery root, if available
   (if not, 3 to 4 celery branches (i.e., pascal))
1 medium parsley root (rarely available; may be omitted)
2 small or one large leek (if not available, use 2 small onions instead)
2 medium onions
garlic to taste
   (may also be squeezed raw into the hot soup instead of cooking it)
small amount of parsley
1-1/2 pounds tomatoes (or more, if desired)
1 pound potatoes

Wash and scrub vegetables and cut into slices or 1/2-inch cubes. Put in large pot, add water to just cover vegetables, bring to a boil, then cook slowly on low heat for 1-1/2 to 2 hours until all the vegetables are soft. Pass through a food mill to remove fibers. Let soup cool before storing in refrigerator.

Please note: **Many spices are high in aromatic acids, which are irritants and are likely to counteract the healing reaction.** This is why only the following mild spices are permitted, to be used in *very small doses*: **allspice, anise, bay leaves, coriander, dill, fennel, mace, marjoram, rosemary, saffron, sage, sorrel, summer savory, tarragon and thyme. In addition, chives, garlic, onion and parsley may be used in larger amounts. Two herb teas—chamomile and peppermint—are frequently used by Gerson patients.** For details, please see Chapter 18, "All About Enemas," p. 155, and Chapter 20, "Understanding Healing Reactions," p. 171.

All About Enemas

T o the uninitiated, the coffee enema is the most surprising and apparently bizarre element of the Gerson Therapy. Critics like to attack and ridicule it without bothering to find out its purpose and function. **Yet, without this simple tool of detoxification, the Gerson method wouldn't work.** Before going into details, let us make clear why this is so.

The moment a patient is put on the full therapy, the combined effect of the food, the juices and the medication causes the immune system to flush out accumulated toxins from the body tissues. This great clearing-out procedure carries the risk of over-burdening and poisoning the liver— the all-important organ of detoxification, which is bound to be already damaged and debilitated.

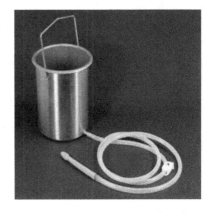

Generally speaking, any kind of enema introduces a substance into the rectum in order to empty the bowel or to administer nutrients or drugs. **It is a medical procedure of great antiquity.** Hippocrates, the

Greek "father of modern medicine," prescribed water enemas for several conditions some 2,600 years ago. In India, enemas were recommended for inner cleansing by Patanjali, author of the first written work on yoga, in around 200 B.C. According to tradition, the ibis (a sacred bird of ancient Egypt associated with wisdom) used to administer itself an enema with its long curved beak.

Closer to our own time, a lady in the court of King Louis XIV of France is reported to have taken an enema under her voluminous skirts, and "Le Malade Imaginaire" (i.e., "The Hypochondriac," in Moliere's play of the same title) enjoyed an enema on stage. It is only in recent times, and mainly in English-speaking countries, that this simple and safe cleansing method had fallen into disuse.

The use of coffee as enema material began in Germany towards the end of World War I (1914–1918). The country was blockaded by the Allies and many essential goods—among them, morphine—were not available, yet trainloads of wounded soldiers kept arriving at field hospitals, needing surgery. The surgeons had barely enough morphine to dull the pain of the operations but none to help patients endure the postsurgical pain; all they could do was to use water enemas.

Although, owing to the blockade, coffee was in short supply, there was plenty of it around to help the surgeons stay awake during their long spells of duty. The nurses, desperate to ease their patients' pain, began to pour some of the leftover coffee into the enema buckets. They figured that, since it helped the surgeons (who drank it), the soldiers (who didn't) would also benefit from it. Indeed, the soldiers reported pain relief.

This accidental discovery came to the attention of two medical researchers—Professors Meyer and Huebner at the University of Goettingen[1] in Germany—who went on to test the effects of rectally infused caffeine on rats. **They found that the caffeine, traveling via the hemorrhoidal vein and the portal system to the liver, opened up the bile ducts, allowing the liver to release accumulated toxins.** This observation was confirmed 70 years later, in 1990, by Peter Lechner, MD,[2] oncologist surgeon at the District Hospital of Graz, Austria, after running a six-year controlled test on cancer patients following a slightly modified version of the Gerson Therapy. **In his report, he quotes independent laboratory results, identifying the two components of coffee that play the major role in detoxifying the liver.** (See Chapter 12, "Why Does the Gerson Therapy Work?," p. 111.)

Dr. Gerson became aware of the benefits of enemas early in developing his treatment, and they have remained a cornerstone of his therapy to this day. It is important to realize that, while the patient is holding the coffee enema in his or her colon for the suggested 12 to 15 minutes, the body's entire blood supply passes through the liver every three minutes (i.e., four to five times in all), carrying poisons picked up from the tissues. These are then released through the bile ducts due to the stimulation of the caffeine.

However, in order to leave the body, these toxins still have to travel through the small intestine (25 to 27 feet), through the colon (4 to 5 feet) and out via the rectum and the anus. Naturally, on this long trip, a small amount of the released toxins is reabsorbed into the system and can cause the patient discomfort, especially in the early phase of the therapy, when detoxification had only just started. This is the reason why, in the beginning, five or more enemas are taken daily.

Important warning: **Although high colonics have become fashionable among some celebrities, they must not be used by Gerson patients.** Dr. Gerson had stated this very clearly, and we can only reiterate his conclusion. In high colonics, up to 5 quarts of water are forced into the whole length of the large intestine, under pressure that can easily distend it. When the water is released, it washes out the fluids, enzymes, minerals and other nutrients from the colon, together with the friendly bacteria which are vital for good digestion. This can increase the risk of a mineral imbalance. On the other hand, high colonics don't serve the all-important reason for the use of coffee enemas, namely the opening of the bile ducts, which helps the liver to release toxins and cleanse itself. **On no account should anyone make the mistake of thinking that high colonics are interchangeable with coffee enemas.**

We have presented the history and theoretical background. Now let us the practicalities.

The Basics of Preparing and Performing a Coffee Enema and Using the Equipment

The basic components of the coffee enema are the following:

- Organic, medium or light roast drip-grind coffee
- Filtered, or if from a fluoridated source, distilled water
- Enema equipment

The current price of an enema bucket ranges from $40 to $60. The equipment must be carefully chosen, as not all products on the market are suitable. The earliest type—the combination syringe—is a rubber hot-water bottle, complete with appropriate tubing and rectal or vaginal tip. This works well for occasional use or travel but it is difficult to clean. Other rubber bags, not "combination syringes," have a much wider opening, which makes them easier to clean. However, they don't stand up well to constant use.

Most popular among Gerson patients is the plastic bucket, which has an easy-to-read register of ounces. This shows how much of the coffee the patient has introduced into the rectum. The bucket is easy to clean and has only one drawback: if dropped or cleaned too vigorously, it can break and must be replaced.

That risk is avoided by choosing a stainless steel bucket, now available at the relatively cheap price of about $30, including the needed attachments. It is unbreakable and easy to clean, even with very hot water, which shouldn't be used with the plastic bucket. The rubber tubing needs to be replaced occasionally. The only disadvantage of this type is that, not being transparent, one cannot check how far the enema process has progressed.

The standard mixture for one enema consists of 3 rounded tablespoons of organic, medium or light roast drip-grind coffee and 4 cups (1 quart or 32 ounces) of filtered or distilled water. The procedure is to bring the water to a boil, add the coffee, let it boil for 3 minutes, then turn down the heat and let it simmer (covered) for 15 minutes. Let it cool, then strain it through a cloth-lined strainer. (A piece of clean, white linen or nylon can be used.) Check the amount left after straining and replace the water that has boiled away to restore it to 1 quart.

For patients on the therapy, it is best to prepare the whole day's requirement at once rather than cooking each portion separately every 4 hours. In other words, a coffee concentrate is produced, saving much time and effort. Take a pot which holds at least 3 quarts, put in about 2 quarts of filtered or distilled water, bring it to a boil and add 15 rounded tablespoons of coffee, which will be enough for five enemas, then proceed as above. After straining the liquid, take five 1-quart jars or juice bottles, pour the same amount of the concentrate into each, then add enough water to make up the volume to 8 ounces of concentrate.

The standard mixture for one enema (i.e., 8 ounces of coffee concentrate and 24 ounces of water, making a total of 32 ounces) has to be warmed to body temperature and poured into the enema bucket, having first clamped the tube shut to stop the liquid from running out. Before starting the enema, a small amount of the solution should be released to clear the tube of air. It is a good idea to eat a small piece of fruit to get the digestive system going, especially before the first morning enema. This will provide a little glucose to raise the low blood sugar after a night's sleep.

The more relaxed the patient is, the easier the enema experience will be. That requires comfort. Unless a couch or folding camp bed is available, an enema "nest" is made on the bathroom floor, with a large, soft towel or blanket as its base, covered with an enema mat or a soft polyester shower curtain for accidental leaks or spillage and a pillow or cushion for the head. **The bucket is placed at approximately 18 inches above the body, hanging from a hook or standing on a stool. The coffee should not flow in too fast or with too much pressure.** About 2 inches of the tube's tip is lubricated with Vaseline and gently inserted some 8 to 10 inches into the anus, and the clamp on the tube is released to let the coffee flow in. **The patient lies on his or her right side with legs pulled up in the fetal position, relaxed and breathing deeply. When all the coffee is absorbed, it should be held in for 12 to 15 minutes, before evacuating.**

Many patients enjoy the relaxed comfort of enema time—**"upside-down coffee,"** as some call it—and use it to listen to soothing music, to meditate or to read. One young lady, recovering from a brain tumor on the Gerson program over some two years, first read all the main classics, then switched to philosophy, followed by mathematics, and subsequently became so well read that she won a top scholarship! She also made a full recovery.

How Many? How Often?

Most patients with bone and joint diseases can do with two or three enemas a day. Unless they are seriously ill with kidney problems, nonhealing skin lesions and sores or gangrene of the extremities, they can use a somewhat easier therapy. If the problems are more severe, they will do better, respond faster and heal with a stricter approach.

In such cases, more juices (eight to 10 glasses a day) and more enemas (four to five a day) are suggested. It is important to remember that juice intake has to be adjusted to enema use since enemas tend to flush out minerals from the large intestine (causing electrolyte imbalance) unless these are replenished with the intake of juices, high in minerals.

Also remember that coffee enemas do not interfere with the normal activity of the colon, producing daily bowel movements. Occasionally, patients worry about that but their fears are groundless. Once the liver and the digestive system are fully restored, normal elimination takes over, even in those who had previously suffered from constipation.

Possible Problems

Many patients learn the enema routine without difficulty and enjoy the feeling of lightness and added energy yielded by the practice. Others, however, experience difficulties, which need to be addressed. Some of the problems that may arise are listed below.

Patients may arrive at the hospital with a massive accumulation of stool in their colon, caused by the use of heavy pain-killing drugs, including morphine. These tend to paralyze peristalsis (the alternate contraction and relaxation of the intestine, by which the contents are propelled onward), causing severe constipation. As a result, these patients are unable to take in a quart (32 ounces) of the coffee solution, let alone hold it in. The answer for them is to take whatever amount they can comfortably accommodate, stop and hold this as long as possible (even if only for a few minutes), then release and take the remaining coffee solution. Again, hold it and release after 12 to 15 minutes. As a rule, after two or three days, when the colon has been cleared of old accumulations, the whole enemas can be taken and held without difficulty.

Some patients may suffer from gas retention, which stops the enema from getting into the colon. When that happens, a small amount—say 6 to 10 ounces—of the coffee can be infused, after which the bucket is lowered to the patient's level, allowing the coffee to flow back into the bucket. This often releases the gas, causing some "bubbling" in the bucket. The bucket is then raised again and, after the clearing of the gas, the enema can continue more easily.

The patient is supposed to take the enema lying on his or her right side in order to help the coffee solution get into the transverse colon from the descending colon. However, as a result of surgery or arthritis, the right side may be painful. In such a case, the patient can lie on his or her back, with their legs pulled up, and proceed from that position.

If a patient suffers from severe irritation of the colon, a small portion of the coffee concentrate, say 2 to 4 ounces, can be diluted with chamomile tea instead of water. The smaller amount of coffee will still help to detoxify the liver while the chamomile tea soothes the colon. There is no time limit for the use of chamomile tea. **In the case of severe diarrhea, an enema of chamomile tea only is used for gentle morning and evening cleansing.**

To prepare chamomile tea, put 1 ounce of the dried flower heads into a glass dish, add 1 pint of boiling water, cover the dish and let it stand in a warm place to infuse for 15 minutes. Strain, cool and store it in a stoppered bottle for a maximum of three days. Increase amounts in the above proportion as required. Chamomile is one of the herbs most used in the Gerson Therapy, both as an enema component and as an herbal drink.

Sometimes a patient has been doing enemas for the first few days of the treatment without a problem, but suddenly he or she cannot get more than 8 to 12 ounces into the colon. This may be a symptom of a healing reaction or flare-up, and the solution is to take what is possible, release it and take the rest. Even if the coffee solution has to be infused in three small amounts, it doesn't matter.

Flare-ups are dealt with in detail in Chapter 20, "Understanding Healing Reactions," p. 171. In brief, they occur when so much bile is released that the intestine is unable to contain it all. The bile then overflows and backs up into the stomach. Since the stomach needs to be acid in order to hold and digest food, the highly alkaline bile produces enormous discomfort; the stomach cannot hold food or liquid and the patient vomits. In itself, this type of flare-up is welcome because it clears out a lot of toxic bile but, in the process, the stomach membrane becomes irritated and needs instant relief. **To do that, the patient needs to drink as much peppermint tea and oatmeal gruel (see Chapter 20) as possible.** At the same time, the coffee enemas are reduced since they are causing the heavy flow of bile. The correct order for the next two to three days is two chamomile enemas and only one coffee enema a day, until the nausea and vomiting clear up. Then the regular schedule can be resumed.

During the flare-up, if the patient vomits and also has diarrhea, the body loses a lot of fluid, so dehydration must be prevented.

One way is to use more chamomile enemas instead of coffee. Also, the apple/carrot and green juices can be used as rectal implants. The regular 8-ounce dose of juice is warmed to body temperature by placing the glass in a warm water bath (not on the stove and without diluting it) and gently infused into the rectum. **This is not an enema and the patient should hold it until the liquid is absorbed.** That may not take more than 10 to 15 minutes of lying still in bed. These infusions can be used with all the juices (except orange and grapefruit) every hour, instead of having them as drinks—particularly valuable at times when, during the flare-up, the patient cannot even bear to look at a juice, let alone drink it.

Another problem occurs when the patient takes in the full 32 ounces of coffee solution but, after 12 minutes, is unable to release it. When that happens, the usual reaction is to take another enema, expecting it to push out the first lot, but that doesn't happen and the patient tends to panic. The reason for the blockage is that the colon spasms, cramps and doesn't release the liquid. Of course, there is no danger in this—the colon could actually hold up to 5 quarts—but that is not the point. If the trouble is caused by cramping, the patient needs to lie down on his or her side, with a warm water bottle on their stomach, and try to relax. If the situation lasts a little longer, including the time for the next enema, it helps to put 2 tablespoons of the regular potassium compound (see Chapter 19, "Medications," p. 165) into each enema for a few days. This will help to release cramps and/or spasms.

Please note: **Do not use this method for more than two to three days to avoid irritating the rectum and the colon.**

It is only when they are on the regular enema routine that patients realize how much waste material their bodies have stored over many years. Once the organism gets a go-ahead in the direction of self-cleansing, it does release a variety of strange, disturbing accumulations which appear in the enema returns, including a wide range of parasites. Experts claim that some 85% of us harbor parasites in our colon, which are best expelled. So the message is not to panic **if the enema returns contain unusual substances; they prove that detoxification and cleansing is progressing well.**

Cleaning the Equipment

Like all other tools of the Gerson program, the enema bucket has to be kept clean. Since the anus, rectum and colon are not sterile, the equipment need not be sterilized. After each use, the bucket has to be rinsed with hot, soapy water, running it through the tube as well, and then rinsed again thoroughly to remove the soap. **Two or three times a week, it is wise to put a cup of 3% hydrogen peroxide (from the super-**

market or drug store) into the bucket with the clamp closed and let it stand overnight to kill any germs or impurities. Rinse it out before the first use in the morning.

CAUTION

If you keep the plastic tube attached to the bucket, it will eventually become loose and even slip off, treating you to an unwanted coffee shower. Check the fit frequently and, if necessary, cut an inch or so from the loosened end of the tube and replace the tight part. You can prevent accidents by removing the plastic tube every time before running hot water through the bucket, so that it shrinks back to its original size and remains tightly in position.

REFERENCES

1. M. Gerson, *A Cancer Therapy: Results of Fifty Cases and The Cure of Advanced Cancer by Diet Therapy: A Summary of Thirty Years of Clinical Experimentation,* 6th ed. (San Diego, CA: Gerson Institute, 1999).
2. Peter Lechner, MD, "Dietary Regime to be Used in Oncological Postoperative Care," Proceedings of the Oesterreicher Gesellschaft fur Chirurgie (Jun. 21-23, 1984).

CHAPTER 19

Medications

F or the general public, "medications" normally mean drugs, used in allopathic medicine in the treatment of disease. In acute cases and emergencies, many drugs are life saving and highly valuable. However, when it comes to chronic conditions, as a rule, the synthetic drugs, which are alien to the body, can merely alleviate (i.e., suppress) symptoms without dealing with the basic cause. This process is often accompanied by severe side effects, which may require more drugs to control.

The medications used in the Gerson Therapy belong to a totally different category. Far from being drugs, they are nutritional supplements consisting of natural substances present in, and needed for, the normal functioning of the various body systems. Being natural, they have no damaging side effects. Their purpose is to make up for the deficiencies of the sick body until it recovers sufficiently to cover all its needs. These substances are so pure that, even if they are incorrectly used by mistake or are in excessive or insufficient doses, they do no harm—with the exception of the thyroid/iodine supplementation, which must be correctly adjusted.

Let us take them one by one and explore their purpose.

Potassium Compound

Dr. Gerson found that the basic problem in all chronic degenerative diseases is the loss of potassium from, and the penetration of sodium into, the cells, now known as the tissue damage syndrome. The average diet in most countries, especially in the developed world, contains far too much salt (sodium), which eventually causes the breakdown of the healthy balance within the body.[1] To correct this, Dr. Gerson added a large amount of potassium (a 10% solution of three potassium salts) to the already potassium-rich, organic vegetarian diet, and observed that this enabled the sick body to release the excess sodium, together with edema, while also reducing high blood pressure and, in most cases, pain.

To prepare the compound, 100 grams of three ready-mixed potassium salts are dissolved in 1 quart of distilled water and stored in a dark glass bottle, or in a clear one kept inside a large brown or black paper bag, to keep out all light. On the full intensive therapy, 4 teaspoons of the potassium compound are added to 10 of the freshly prepared fruit and/or vegetable juices. This dosage is reduced after three to four weeks to 2 teaspoons in each of 10 juices.

In seriously ill patients, it takes many months, even one to two years, to restore normal potassium content to the essential organs. The serum potassium level, as shown in the blood test result, does not reflect the potassium status of the cell. Low serum potassium values may signify healing because the depleted tissues are reabsorbing potassium, while high figures may be found in failures because the tissues lose it.

Thyroid and Lugol's Solution

It is a fact—known since Dr. Gerson's day—that most chronically ill patients are suffering from a low basal metabolism.[2] Much of the problem is caused by the chlorine,[3] widely used in the purification of the water supply and, worse still, by fluoride.[4] **Both remove iodine from the thyroid gland,** thus reducing its ability to function properly. The thyroid gland regulates the metabolic rate of the organism, acting as its thermostat, being capable of raising temperature and producing fever. It also affects the immune system as well as the proper functioning of all hormone systems. In high blood pressure caused by atherosclerosis, low metabolism slows the burning of fats, encouraging narrowing of the arteries.

When thyroid and iodine in the form of 1/2 strength Lugol's solution are added to the patient's intake, the immune system becomes reactivated and healing can begin. The patient can start with the doses outlined in Table 21-1, "Schedule for Nonmalignant Patients" in Chapter 21, "The Gerson Therapy for Nonmalignant Diseases," p. 178, and be monitored by a trained Gerson doctor. Thyroid hormone levels may also determined by the patient directly using blood chemistry tests ordered from Direct Labs (www.directlabs.com). This confidential laboratory testing service offers a private and secure online portal where you can order your test and retrieve your results at a very reasonable cost.

The process is simple:

1.   Contact Direct Labs to open an account, complete the necessary authorizations and order your test.

2.   You will then choose a local laboratory that will draw your blood.

3.   In 24 to 48 hours, you will receive an email letting you know that you may log in to your account to view or print your results.

Niacin

Niacin (common name for nicotinic acid, or vitamin B_3) assists in the digestion of protein and helps to open capillary circulation, thus bringing freshly oxygenated blood (from the constant intake of fresh juices) to all body tissues. By improving circulation, it also works to reduce ascites (an abdominal edema where excess water is retained in the abdomen) and pain. The dosage is a 50 mg tablet five times daily, taken during meals. This medication often causes the well-known "niacin flush," a temporary reddening of the face and upper chest area, with some itching. This is totally harmless and passes quickly. (**Do not switch to non-**

flushing niacin; it is ineffective.) Niacin should be discontinued during women's periods or in case of bleeding of any kind.

Liver Capsules

The severely toxic and damaged liver needs maximum assistance to improve its vital functions. The therapy provides this help in the form of liver capsules containing dried, defatted, powdered liver from healthy animals. Two capsules of liver powder are given three times a day with carrot-only juice. According to Dr. Virginia Livingston,[5] the combination of dry liver powder with carrot juice produces abscisic acid, a precursor of vitamin A.

Crude Liver Injections with B$_{12}$ Supplement

Since most chronic disease patients are also anemic (a condition that develops when your blood lacks enough healthy red blood cells), additional vitamin B$_{12}$ is needed to help restore the hemoglobin content of the blood, promoting the formation and maturation of red blood cells. It works against different types of anemia and even against degenerative changes in the spinal cord. As seen in animal experiments, this vitamin is able to restore a wide range of tissues damaged by age, chronic illness, surgery, degenerative diseases or various kinds of poisoning. Intramuscular liver extract (3 cc) with added 50 mcg of B$_{12}$—a tiny amount, a 20th of 1 cc—is given every other day. The frequency is reduced as patient shows recovery.

Pancreatin

This is an extract of various pancreatic digestive enzymes, normally needed to digest fats, proteins and sugar. Gerson patients don't consume those substances; however, these enzymes are vitally important in the digestion and elimination of atherosclerosis. The dosage is 3 tablets of 325 mg each four times a day—one after each meal, plus an additional dose in mid-afternoon.

Acidol Pepsin

This can be used if the patient has a poor appetite since it helps with digestion. **No acidol is given in cases of acid reflux, stomach ulcers, or other irritation of the stomach.**

Flaxseed Oil

Also known as food-grade linseed oil, this contains both essential fatty acids—linoleic acid and linolenic acid—and is particularly rich in the Omega-3 series, as discovered by Johanna Budwig, PhD.[6] The therapeutic effects of flaxseed oil include the following:

- It attracts oxygen at the cell membrane and transports oxygen into the cell.

- It is able to detoxify fat-soluble toxins and helps to dissolve and remove plaque.

- It is a carrier of vitamin A, which is important for the immune system.

- It removes excess cholesterol, an important function, since patients' cholesterol levels sometimes rise during the initial stages of the therapy.

The dose is 2 tablespoons daily for the first month, then 1 tablespoon daily for the rest of the treatment (limited, similar to medications, and reduced to 1 tablespoon daily after 30 days).

Coenzyme Q10

Recently added to the protocol, this coenzyme is valuable in replacing some of the nutrients that were available in the discontinued raw liver juice. It must be administered cautiously at first, since some patients are hypersensitive to this substance. To start, the dose is 50 mg daily for five to seven days, then increased to 100 mg per day, to reach 500 to 600 mg daily.

REFERENCES

1. Freeman Widener Cope, *Physiological Chemistry and Physics* 10 (5) (1978).
2. Kathy Page, "Hypothyroidism and Cancer," supplementary memorandum, UK Parliament Select Committee on Science and Technology (June 2000).
3. Joseph M. Price, *Coronaries, cholesterol, chlorine* (Salem, MA: Pyramid Books, 1971).
4. P. M. Galetti and G. Joyet, "Effect of fluorine on thyroidal iodine metabolism in hyperthyroidism," *Journal of Clinical Endocrinology and Metabolism* 18 (10) (October 1958): 1102-10.
5. Personal communication from Dr. Livingston to Charlotte Gerson (February 1977).
6. Johanna Budwig, PhD, *Flax Oil As a True Aid Against Arthritis Heart Infarction Cancer and Other Diseases,* 3d ed. (Ferndale, WA: Apple Publishing, December 1994).

CHAPTER 20

Understanding Healing Reactions

Healing reactions, also known as flare-ups, are an essential part of the Gerson Therapy. It is important that patients understand their nature and function before embarking on the full treatment, since healing reactions are somewhat paradoxical experiences: although they can produce a number of unpleasant symptoms, they should be welcomed as evidence that the therapy has kicked in and is working well.

Let's see how and when this necessary process is likely to begin. As a rule, after the first few days on the full Gerson program, the patients feel better. Naturally they are greatly encouraged. That is the moment to remind them that a healing reaction may be on the way and to explain how it is going to promote detoxification. Without proper preparation, the sudden shift is hard to bear!

Arthritic patients are usually less severely ill than those with diabetes, high blood pressure, cancer, etc., due to the highly toxic medications the latter are taking. Nevertheless, both patients and doctors need to understand that the entire public eating the "standard American diet" has accumulated a level of toxicity, no matter what their diagnosis or disease—even if they are not sick! Therefore, as the Gerson Therapy begins to work, the fatty tissue dissolves and releases toxic materials the body has stored there!

In addition, when the reactions start, the calcium deposits in the arteries (atherosclerosis) are released into the bloodstream and could cause clots. This does not happen when the therapy is faithfully practiced. The regimen should not be changed during such a flare-up or "healing reaction." This protects the patient and we have observed no sudden clotting (heart attacks or strokes). No blood-thinning drugs should be needed.

Again, the patient must be prepared for these reactions, which may be accompanied by toxic stools, lack of appetite and even aversion to food or drink, especially to the green juices. There can also be more gas than usual, plus difficulties with the coffee enemas (due to increased toxic pressure from the liver). **Without advance warning, the patients may feel that their condition is worsening.**

The first flare-up is usually relatively short, since the body is not yet able to carry out serious healing in its weakened condition and is only just beginning to respond. Even that early start can produce impressive results. The body begins to heal old injuries, fractures, lumpy scars and serious conditions, including long-standing high blood pressure and age-onset diabetes. **This process cannot be held back or stopped since the body is not able to heal selectively!** In other words, it does not only heal the present life-threatening disease but also clears up all other damage, whether old or new. That is what the totality of the Gerson Therapy means. Thanks to it, patients have overcome allergies, long-term migraines, arthritis, fibromyalgia and other conditions that have troubled them for any length of time.

How do patients react to a flare-up? Only a general answer can be given based on the reactions of a majority of cases. Since each person is different and has a different medical past with different damages to the body, each healing reaction is also different. It is also impossible to give an exact answer to patients who wish to know how long a flare-up will last. In many cases, the first reaction is mild and only lasts from a few hours to a day or two. The second one is normally longer and somewhat heavier, since the body and its immune system have, to some extent, been detoxified, strengthened with the enzymes and nutrients contained in the raw juices and supported by the medication. As a result, it is able to respond more powerfully.

What should one do for the patient in a flare-up who is unwell, upset and dismayed? One should not stop the therapy and give no coffee enemas or juices, for doing so would drastically stop the healing process, yet we must help the patient to endure the discomforts of the flare-ups. Here are the best ways:

Nausea

If, despite the nausea, the patient is able to drink the juices, by all means continue to provide them. If he or she develops a severe aversion to the green juice, warm it gently (undiluted) to body temperature by standing the container in a warm water bath, pour the juice into the enema bucket and infuse it rectally as a retention implant. **This is not an enema and should not be expelled.**

The patient should lie comfortably in bed, with legs pulled up in the fetal position, and allow the juice to be absorbed. Patients who are temporarily unable to drink any juices can have them administered rectally (all except the orange juice) and should be encouraged to drink warm oatmeal gruel and plenty of peppermint tea, partly to settle the stomach and also to supply the necessary liquids which would normally be provided by the juices.

To prepare oatmeal gruel, place 1 ounce of oats and 5 ounces of water into a pot and bring to a boil. Let it simmer for 10 to 15 minutes, then strain through a fine tea strainer to remove all solids. Press the oats as far as possible through the strainer in order to obtain a liquid somewhat denser than water. Drink while warm.

For patients severely sensitive to juices during a flare-up, 2 ounces of gruel can be poured into a glass and topped with no more than 6 ounces of juice.

Peppermint tea helps to relieve nausea, digestive discomfort and gas. Peppermint or spearmint is easy to grow in the backyard and spreads quickly. A heaped tablespoon of fresh leaves makes one cup of tea; add boiling distilled water, cover and let it steep for 12 to 15 minutes, then strain. If you use tea bags, make sure they are organic. One tea bag easily makes two cups. If you buy loose leaves, which is preferable, put a tablespoon of leaves in the pot, pour 2 cups of boiling distilled water over them, and proceed as above.

It is a good idea to leave peppermint tea in a thermos on the patient's bedside table, in case he or she wakes up thirsty at night.

Controlling Diarrhea

- Stop all juices. Give the patient frequent cups of peppermint tea, at least 5 or 6 daily. Add 1/8 teaspoon of potassium gluconate powder (**not the potassium compound**) in every cup.

- Food should consist of oatmeal 3 times per day, with brown sugar (no honey) and applesauce.

- Suspend coffee enemas. Use only chamomile tea enemas 2-3 times per day.

- Restart coffee enemas when condition improves. It is best to restart enemas using camomile tea to dilute the coffee concentrate.

- As the intestinal tract calms down, gradually start juices. Place 2-3 ounces of oatmeal gruel into each cup, then add 5-6 ounces of juice. Do not add any medication. Avoid salads for 1-2 days. Continue oatmeal with applesauce.

- When juices are tolerated, add medication.

- Gradually reduce peppermint tea.

- Appetite may be temporarily reduced but will return later. Meanwhile, raw foods are better tolerated than cooked dishes. However, if patient prefers, he/she can use soup, potatoes (without eating the skin) and some cooked, soft vegetables.

- You can give 2 charcoal tablets, ground up in tea, after each loose bowel movement. This helps to absorb and reduce gas or other discomfort.

- If diarrhea lasts for more than 3 days, the stool specimen should be tested. However, diarrhea is mostly one of the symptoms of the healing reaction.

Depression

Dr. Gerson notes[1] that it is not unusual for the patient to be depressed, temporarily during a flare-up. Such emotional outbursts run parallel with the body's attempts to detoxify: **remember the mind and body are connected and cannot be separated.**

Often, an extra enema helps to ease the upheaval. The patient may even pick a fight with the caregiver for no obvious reason. This is less surprising if we consider the metabolic fact that aggression produces extra adrenalin, which makes the person actually feel better! The caregiver should not be hurt by any unwarranted attacks or accusations. The patient cannot control these outbursts and usually regrets them afterwards. Again, a coffee enema can clear the problem. This part of the healing reaction should be seen as a psychological cleansing. Once the flare-up is over, the patient will again be optimistic and forward-looking.

REFERENCE

1. M. Gerson, *A Cancer Therapy: Results of Fifty Cases and The Cure of Advanced Cancer by Diet Therapy: A Summary of Thirty Years of Clinical Experimentation,* 6th ed. (San Diego, CA: Gerson Institute, 1999), pp. 201-202.

CHAPTER 21

The Gerson Therapy for Nonmalignant Diseases

F rom his long clinical practice, Dr. Gerson was able to establish that a patient suffering from a nonmalignant disease had a sick, damaged liver, while the liver of someone with a malignancy was severely toxic (poisoned). Based on this difference, he adjusted the treatment accordingly, creating a less-intensive therapy for nonmalignant conditions. At the same time, he specified that, if patients in the latter category followed a stricter protocol closely resembling the full intensive therapy, they recovered faster.

The less-intensive therapy is less demanding and easier to follow, so that patients on this regime can continue working. This is a great advantage since most people depend on their earned income and cannot leave their jobs for any length of time. Table 21-1 is a typical hour-by-hour schedule for patients on the less-intensive therapy.

Note for Table 21-1

- Make yourself a blank schedule to be filled in later as the medications change and the frequency of enemas is reduced.

Table 21-1
SCHEDULE FOR NONMALIGNANT PATIENT

	Enema	Meal	Flaxseed Oil (tbsp.)	Acidol Pepsin Capsules	Juice	Potassium Compound (tsp.)	Lugol's Solution (1/2 Strength) (drops)	Thyroid (gr.)	Niacin (mg.)	Liver Capsules	Pancreatin Tablets	Liver and B$_{12}$ Injection
8:00 a.m.		Breakfast		2	Orange	2	1	1	50	2	3	
9:00 a.m.	Coffee				Green	2						
10:00 a.m.					Carrot/apple	2			50			
11:00 a.m.					Carrot					2		Every 2nd day
12:00 p.m.					Green	2						
1:00 p.m.		Lunch	1	2	Carrot/apple	2	1	1	50		3	
2:00 p.m.	Coffee				Green	2						
5:00 p.m.					Carrot/apple	2			50		3	
6:00 p.m.	Coffee				Green	2						
7:00 p.m.		Dinner	1	2	Carrot/apple	2	1		50	2	3	

It is difficult to specify the amount of time it may take for patients to reduce the intensity of the treatment. It depends on the degree of damage, their ability to heal, their age, encouragement and help in the home, and possible psychological factors. Often, the patient knows when the time is right. Nonetheless, it is important not to discontinue the treatment too soon or too abruptly. Serious problems could result.

CHAPTER 22

Things to Remember

I n this chapter, we present a number of miscellaneous items in support of your efforts to improve and protect your health. Knowledge is power, and the emergence of the so-called "expert patient" around the world is a sure sign that more and more people are willing to take responsibility for their health and well-being. No doubt you are one of them. We hope you will find the following information useful.

Complementary Therapies

These days, there is a bewildering array of complementary treatments offered and the question arises whether Gerson patients should use any of these. The simple answer is that anything which promotes healing and does not clash with the requirements of the therapy is permissible and potentially helpful. However, there is little margin for error, so let us review which techniques are safe to use.

Reflexology or Zone Therapy

This dates back to ancient Egypt, China and India. **It is based on the principle that the feet and hands are a mirror image of the body** and that, by applying pressure to certain points— especially on the feet—corresponding parts of the body are affected. The purpose of the treatment is to break up congestion, blockages and patterns of stress and restore homeostasis, the 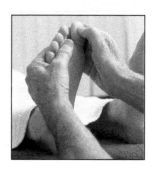 body's internal equilibrium. Reflexology does not claim to diagnose or cure, but it has a good record of improving general well-being.

Reiki

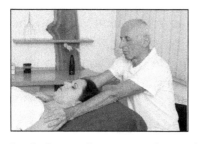

This is a Japanese technique for stress reduction and relaxation that promotes healing. **Its practitioners claim that there is an invisible life-force energy that flows through us and keeps us alive.** If this energy becomes low, we fall sick and suffer from stress. In order to heal, the Reiki master channels the energy through his or her hands into the patient's body. There is no need for massage, only for very gentle touch. Although the patient feels very little, the treatment is truly holistic, affecting body, emotions, mind and spirit. Because of its nonspecific nature, Reiki is able to help in any disease and works well with other medical or therapeutic techniques. The word itself consists of two parts: *Rei* means higher power and *Ki* stands for life-force energy, so the implication is that Reiki is a spiritually guided way of restoring universal life-force energy in those who need it.

Acupuncture

This originated in China some 2,000 years ago and has been known and increasingly practiced in the United States since 1971. Its essence is the stimulation of certain anatomical points on the body by penetrating the skin with thin metal nee- 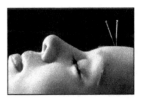 dles and manipulating them by hand or electrical means. This is claimed to regulate the nervous system, activate the body's own painkilling biochemicals and strengthen the immune system. Acupuncture has a proven record of good pain control and of hastening recovery from surgery. It can impart a sense of well-being and boosts depleted energy. Acupuncture needles, which cause minimal pain, were approved by the Food and Drug Administration for use by licensed practitioners in 1996.[1] Today, this ancient technique is used in the United States by thousands of physicians, dentists and other practitioners for the prevention or relief of pain.

Yoga

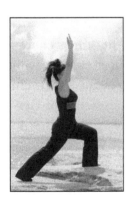

Yoga first emerged in India some 5,000 years ago. It has several varieties, including hatha yoga, a physical discipline consisting mainly of stretching and breathing exercises, which has grown in popularity in the West since the mid-20th century. Being noncompetitive, gentle and accessible to people of all ages and levels of ability, yoga is an ideal exercise for Gerson patients who wish to improve their flexibility, stamina and muscle tone.

Yoga postures, known as asanas, help to achieve balance and poise. The breathing exercises are soothing and relaxing and increase the supply of oxygen to the organism.

Chi Gung

Ancient Chinese teachings advise that vital life force energy—also known as "chi"—flows through your body in specific channels or rivers called "meridians." When the meridians are open and flowing properly, the body is strong and healthy. When the meridians are obstructed or chi flow is blocked, health wanes, resulting in sickness and disease.

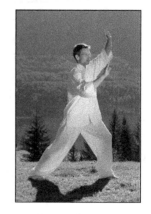

Interestingly, there is some agreement between Dr. Gerson's reasons for poor health and the principles of chi gung (pronounced *chee-gung*) regarding blocked chi flow. They both may result from poor diet, toxicity, a sedentary lifestyle and stress.

While chi gung is relatively new in Western society, quite a bit of research has been done in the East supporting its health benefits. Millions of people around the world practice chi gung every day because they say it makes them healthier, boosts their energy and helps them feel better.

Practitioners of chi gung learn to strengthen their life-force energy and open their meridians by combining slow body movements with deep-breathing techniques and mental visualizations that cause their chi to move throughout the body. Chi gung is an excellent exercise for Gerson patients of all ages as it is done in a relaxed manner and creates no pain or stress in your body.

REFERENCE

1. "Get the Facts: Acupuncture," National Center for Complementary and Alternative Medicine (http://nccam.nih.gov/health/acupuncture).

CHAPTER 23

Watch Out: Pitfalls Ahead!

A s humans, we can make mistakes in any area of life—but when seriously ill people undertake a potentially life-saving program, such as the Gerson Therapy, even a minor blunder or oversight could cause a setback. This way of healing demands a total transformation—not only of lifestyle but also of how the patients understand the principles of sickness, health and healing, and how they respond to their bodies' needs. This understanding is all the more important because the therapy forbids a great many things that are normal parts of the Western lifestyle, and patients need to know the reason behind the strictures in order to accept them wholeheartedly.

There is also the matter of observing the rules of the therapy, even without an authority figure to check or chide the patient as there would be in a conventional medical setting. **It takes maturity and inner strength to be one's own supervisor and stay on the straight and narrow path, but the rewards are enormous and make it all more than worthwhile.**

Save Up Your Energy!

Let's take a close look at the possible mistakes, temptations and trip-wires that a patient is likely to encounter, especially in the early stages of the Gerson protocol. Ironically, the first pitfall is the great improvement in the patient's condition that sets in during the first few weeks on the full therapy, especially if these are spent at the Gerson clinic in Mexico.

When such patients return home—and this holds true especially for women—they look and feel better and are often free from pain, so the family assumes that they can once again rely on the patients to take up all "normal" duties and serve them.

- This is a particularly heavy burden on the wife/mother, who probably feels guilty anyway for "letting down" the family by being ill and having very real needs of her own; guilt may drive her back into her normal routine.

- Male patients normally have a more relaxed attitude on coming home, but even they want to start to work, exercise or deal with chores around the house.

- **Neither behavior is acceptable.**

As stated before, patients need a great deal of rest. Their bodies are working hard to detoxify and heal, and that is more important than any domestic activity. Actually, in most cases, although patients look remarkably better, they do feel tired and even weak for the first two to three months of the therapy, unable to indulge in much activity. Instead of listening to their bodies' message, some patients actually force themselves to be up, make their own food and juice (a six- to eight-hour daily job!) and exhaust themselves. That is a serious mistake.

A similar problem arises, three to four months into the therapy, when the initial tiredness goes and energy returns to such an extent that patients feel virtually normal. They want to be fully active again and make up for "lost time."

Women launch themselves into major housecleaning by washing curtains, scrubbing floors and attacking mountains of ironing; men clear out the garage and, according to the season, either shovel snow or cut the lawn, or even repair the roof, just to prove that they are fully functioning once more. The urge is understandable but must be resisted to avoid a sudden downturn. **Superficial improvements (e.g., increased energy) do not equal healing.** Rest and more rest are still essential to avoid a sudden downturn.

One of Dr. Gerson's important rules was that patients should be in bed no later than 10 p.m.—not reading or watching television or listening to the radio—but sleeping, if possible, or at least at complete rest. The time before midnight is particularly valuable for the body's self-repairing and restoring work and must not be curtailed.

Bending the Rules

Admittedly, the dietary rules of the Gerson Therapy are pretty strict and, while most patients quickly get used to them, there are some who long for their now-forbidden favorite foods (never mind that those had probably contributed to their health breakdown!). **These patients tend to think that surely having a "little extra" on the side every now and then can't possibly do much harm, and would even raise their morale and improve their mood.**

This is wrong on all counts. First of all, how much is "a little" and how often is "every now and then"? Furthermore, once the strict adherence to the protocol is broken, it's easy and tempting to break it again … and again. Also consider that, since in this treatment the body receives instructions and messages via precisely calculated nutrients, each of which affects all the others, to disturb the process with occasional additions of salty, fatty, chemical-laden junk food sounds like a disastrous idea.

Often, it is not the patient but well-meaning visitors—friends and relatives—who suggest breaking the diet and having "a nice big steak to build you up!" They are the ones who question how a grown person can survive, let alone heal, on all that "rabbit food" and, even if the patient manages to ignore their advice, a certain irritation ensues. **Please remember that people who criticize the Gerson protocol, including** otherwise helpful and well-meaning health professionals, do so out of ignorance and incomprehension and, for that reason, can be safely ignored. It's best to ask your visitors and friends to please respect your choice of treatment and support and encourage you—or else leave you alone. Ask those who suggest changes to the therapy, "How many patients have you healed with your advice?"

Being Firm with Friendly Doctors

A friendly allopathic doctor willing to support a Gerson patient is a great asset if he or she agrees to prescribe the necessary blood tests and urinalyses. The problem arises when he or she reads the test results. If any item is out of the normal range, the doctor suggests that the patient take some drug or medication "to bring it to the normal level." That, too, can be a serious mistake. The abnormal value will clear up on the Gerson Therapy, but allopathic drugs can cause damage.

For example, we know of a doctor who noticed a somewhat low iron level in the patient's blood and prescribed an iron medication. The trouble is that iron supplements are toxic,[1] which automatically rules them out for Gerson patients. In time, with all the green juices, liver medication and vitamin B_{12}, the blood readings will return to normal without drugs.

Flare-Ups and Mood Swings

Healing reactions or so-called flare-ups are regular events on the Gerson Therapy. (See Chapter 20, "Understanding Healing Reactions," p. 171.) These episodes can be frighteningly intense; at the same time, the patient may also suffer from depression and a black mood. If the family panics, the patient may end up in the emergency room of the nearest hospital, where the doctors are kind and concerned and give the patient a shot or a pill to stop the symptoms. Unfortunately, they also stop the healing, which has caused serious problems in some cases. **The fact is that the average allopathic doctor has probably never heard of a healing reaction, does not understand its symptoms and function and**

therefore can't be expected to handle it correctly. The proper way to deal with a flare-up is clearly set out in Chapter 20 and should be followed closely.

Psychological problems and mood swings are dealt with fully. Here, we only want to acknowledge the power of occasional fits of negativity, when the patient not only feels physically unwell—with nausea, sweating, headache, horror of food and juices and possibly fever—but is also mentally and emotionally crushed. The toxins cruising through the central nervous system and the brain are to blame, but all the patient feels is an urgent wish to stop the therapy, break out of all the restrictions and run away. This is a passing phase. It is wise to find out about it in advance so that, when it arrives, the patient is more or less prepared and snaps out of it faster.

Water Warning

Don't underestimate the importance of ensuring the purity of all the water used in your home. The worst offender is fluoride, so make sure that your water supply is free from this harmful chemical. If it is not, you must take special precautions. **Unlike chlorine, fluoride is not eliminated by boiling the water! The only way to get rid of it is by distillation. (See Chapter 14, "The Gerson Household," p. 123.)**

However, fluoride is also present in the water used for the daily shower. Although a shower needn't take many minutes, even brief exposure to warm water opens the pores, so that any undesirable component in the water gets quickly absorbed. There are two solutions to this problem:

- Take a sponge bath, instead of a shower, in a gallon of warmed distilled water poured into a basin or sink.

- Install a camping shower in the bathroom and fill it with warmed distilled water. Full description, various models and prices of this appliance are available on the Internet.

Mind What You Read

Knowledge is power and the well-informed patient is likely to make the right choices. However, the big and growing range of so-called health books and diet bibles is a dangerous area full of contradictory theories and advice. Open-minded patients keen to learn new things read as many health books as they can find and end up confused. Although most nutritional methods are at least in part based on the Gerson Therapy, none is complete or free from its author's prejudices and subjective ideas.

If you have decided to use the Gerson Therapy, inform yourself about it as thoroughly as you can and stay with it. After all, it has the longest and best track record.

Cutting Corners

No one can deny that the Gerson Therapy is labor-intensive; at times, it can feel truly overwhelming. When that happens, patients and/or their caregivers may feel tempted to ease things a little bit by changing the routine (e.g., by preparing all the day's juices in one go and storing them in the refrigerator, instead of making them fresh every hour on the hour as prescribed). This slows the treatment and may lead to failure since **the all-important enzymes in the freshly made juices have a lifespan of some 20 minutes. After that time has elapsed, the minerals, trace elements and most vitamins may survive in the juices, but the living enzymes and their healing power will have been lost.**

Another temptation occurs when some ingredient of the Gerson program becomes hard to obtain, and the patient decides that something else will do just as well in the short term. Extreme caution is needed in such a situation. For instance, if organic carrots are not available, under no circumstances should nonorganic ones be used for juicing (or eating). Commercially grown carrots are saturated with agrochemicals; scrubbing and peeling them will not remove the poisons. As an emergency measure, organic bottled carrot juice may be used on its own or mixed with organic bottled apple juice, **but it should be**

understood that this substitution must only be a short-term solution and not a matter of routine.

One of the worst examples of substitution concerned a woman patient suffering from a collagen disease, who was doing well on the Gerson program until her supply of organic carrots dried up completely. Rather than search for another source, she and her husband decided to substitute orange juice for the elusive carrots, and so she began to drink up to eight glasses of freshly pressed orange juice a day. This would have been harmful to any Gerson patient; in this case, it was disastrous since citrus fruits are counterindicated in all collagen diseases. Her condition deteriorated drastically.

P.S.

Thomas Jefferson wrote, "The price of freedom is eternal vigilance." **Well, the price of getting well is the same: eternal vigilance to avoid pitfalls, resist temptations and decline unasked-for advice from well-meaning outsiders who don't understand what you are doing.** However, you know what you are doing and why, and that is all that matters.

REFERENCE

1.   Anna E. O. Fisher and Declan P. Naughton, "Iron supplements: the quick fix with long-term consequences," *Nutrition Journal* 3 (2) (Jan. 16, 2004).

CHAPTER 24

Taking the New Lifestyle Seriously

Study nature; its eternal laws will keep you.

—*Max Gerson*

The Gerson Therapy is very different from the so-called "normal lifestyle." This makes it difficult for many people to understand its limitations. However, once they understand the reasons for the rules, it is easier to follow them and not cheat.

If and when the cheating becomes too severe, there will be no healing! If the cheating is only "slight," the healing will be slowed down! Depending on the severity of the patient's condition, it is up to each individual to make this choice: **Adhere to the rules to recover, or do not adhere to the rules and interfere with healing.**

Here are some important things to bear in mind:

- The Gerson Therapy is admittedly work intensive. It is almost impossible for a relatively seriously ill patient to work and do the therapy at home for him- or herself.

- **Get help—if only for a few hours in the morning**—to clean the carrots, apples and greens; to make the soup; to prepare the enema concentrate; and to make some of the juices and clean up the machine.

- *Most important:* **Get help to do the housework!** It should not interfere with the preparation of foods and juices. Even if the patient has improved, feels better and looks well, they cannot be expected to take up their "normal" household work, which may include preparing food, doing laundry, dishes, etc., for the rest of the family. Also remember that most household cleansers are toxic. (See Chapter 14, "The Gerson Household," then "Cleaning Chemicals," p. 130.)

- Aside from a rest period of about one hour after lunch, Dr. Gerson felt strongly that the sleep before midnight is the most important sleep. **Don't let television or other items distract you.** If you can't sleep, listen to soft music (without light) and meditate or otherwise relax.

You will also be bombarded with television, radio and newspaper ads, raving about some new treatment or wonder drug. Drugs—whether doctor prescribed, over the counter, or on the street—are invariably liver toxic. Don't trust the hype. Stay with the things of nature!

CHAPTER 25

Frequently Asked Questions

T he Gerson Therapy is so fundamentally different from the usual pill-popping, symptom-centered approach of orthodox medicine that newcomers to this method of healing find some of its details puzzling. It is important to explain the reasons behind the rules; once understood, they prove to be eminently logical. Here is a random selection of the most frequently asked questions with the appropriate answers.

Q: *Why not steam vegetables for a short while, then use the water at the bottom of the pan in the soup, rather than cook all the life out of the vegetables over a long time?*

A: Dr. Gerson was very specific about using the lowest possible heat for cooking vegetables. High heat—steam is hotter than boiling water—changes the colloidal structure of the nutrients, particularly the proteins but also the minerals, and makes them hard to absorb and assimilate. Dr. Gerson even suggested putting a heat disperser under the pan to keep the heat just high enough to simmer the food slowly until well done.

This method does not "cook the life out of the food." The only nutrients that are damaged are the enzymes, which die in temperatures above 140° F (60° C), but patients get a huge supply of enzymes in the fresh raw juices to make up for that loss. The lower heat preserves protein and mineral structures and some vitamins.

Suggesting that the water remaining in the pan should be used acknowledges that the good nutrients, especially the minerals, have been leached out into the water, leaving the cooked vegetables without nutrients! This explains why steamed vegetables have very little taste. Another reason for cooking food slowly at the lowest possible heat is to provide the patient's intestinal tract with "soft bulk" (well-done fiber) to cushion all the raw foods and juices the patient has to consume.

Q: *What about using a B-complex supplement to keep the B vitamins in balance since we use fairly large amounts of B_3 and B_{12}?*

A: Dr. Gerson states in his book[1] that patients were damaged when he administered vitamins B_1 and B_6 to them. The Gerson protocol, with its huge number of juices and fresh foods, is very well balanced and has no need for supplements.

Q: *When can organic soy products be introduced into the diet?*

A: The short answer is ***never***. Soy products of all kinds (e.g., tofu, flour or sauce) contain a substance that blocks absorption of nutrients, besides having a high fat content. **A great deal of research has proven the toxicity of soy, even when grown organically.** The hype claiming soy's usefulness in preventing breast cancer has turned out to be unsubstantiated and the opposite of truth: soy is likely to stimulate malignancy.[2]

Q: *Proper food combining, not mixing starch and fruit, is supposed to be healthy. Why isn't it used on the therapy?*

A: Food combining is probably useful if applied to the average American diet, which is high in animal proteins and sodium (salt). Since all Gerson foods are vegetarian and all vegetables contain a certain amount of starch, it is neither necessary nor possible to separate those two substances.

Q: *Why not supplement vitamins C and E, which help to boost the immune system? Surely one glass of orange juice a day isn't enough?*

A: It is a general misconception that only orange juice contains vitamin C. This is not so. The juices used in the Gerson program are richer in vitamin C than orange juice, and patients consume them in huge quantities every day. Raw salads and fruit increase the intake even further. **Dr. Gerson insisted that no additional vitamins should be given to patients.** Besides, we have found that pharmaceutically produced synthetic vitamins and minerals are poorly absorbed and can even be harmful.

Q: *Potatoes and tomatoes both belong to the deadly nightshade family and are banned from many dietary regimes. Why are they the most used foods on the therapy?*

A: They are not! The most used items are carrots, apples and greens for juicing. Potatoes are extremely nutritious, high in potassium as well as in protein and easily digestible (much more so than rice). Tomatoes are also valuable as they contain vitamins and minerals, including lycopene—a powerful antioxidant that has been extensively researched in recent years and is reputed to boost immune competence.[3] Other vegetables belonging to the nightshade family, such as green peppers and eggplants, are also used in the diet and have never shown any toxic effects.

Q: *How many flare-ups or healing reactions can a patient normally expect?*

A: There is no "normal" number for these. The body produces them as long as it needs to heal. As a rule, the first healing reaction sets in some six to eight days after starting the intensive treatment; the second one comes usually after about six weeks; the third, which is often the most severe, is generally observed after three to three and one-half months. These timings are not fixed and only suggest that the patient can expect healing reactions at certain intervals, which can vary widely in individual cases.

Q: *Are headaches a good sign?*

A: Certainly not. They may be a symptom of flare-ups, when the body is releasing its overload of toxins. In that case, an additional coffee enema should be taken to speed up the process of detoxification. In some rare cases, the toxicity is so high that an enema does not relieve the headache and one or more additional enemas are needed. In almost all patients, as healing progresses, headaches disappear forever, even if they had been a problem for many years. If headaches recur after the therapy has ended, the chances are that exposure to toxins or unsuitable food has occurred and must be avoided in the future.

Q: *When do patients begin to feel better and have more energy?*

A: Almost all patients, including extremely ill ones, feel better after the first week on the therapy. Pain diminishes, appetite returns and sleep improves. All this adds up to a great psychological boost. It also signals the moment when the patient has to be warned about an impending healing reaction, bringing with it days of feeling unwell. A true rise in energy may occur in three to six months, depending on the age and condition of the patient. At that point, it is most important that the patient continues to rest and doesn't launch into multiple activities! The new energy must be used for healing and nothing else. There will be plenty of time later to build muscles and make up for lost exercise time. Trying to do so too soon can result in a serious setback.

Q: *Are there any circumstances under which a Gerson patient should use antibiotics?*

A: Yes, but such circumstances are rare. Since virtually all medical drugs have a toxic component, **Gerson patients are advised not to take any prescription or nonprescription items.** Antibiotics are the exception. While in general medical practice they have been seriously overused, weakening the immune system[4] and producing resistant bacteria,[5] very occasionally they need to be used by patients whose immune system is seriously weakened.

Since it may take considerable time to restore the patient's immune system, in a case of acute infection, antibiotics are required. We use them to help fight colds and attacks of flu, and patients undergoing dental work should take them as recommended by their dentist. **Of course, antibiotics don't kill viruses, but they can control the opportunistic infections that attack a weakened body.** For colds, we use the least toxic antibiotics, namely penicillin, unless the patient is allergic to it. For other infections, the appropriate antibiotic has to be chosen. For patients on the Gerson Therapy, adding one aspirin, one 500 mg tablet of vitamin C, and 50 mg of niacin, taken together with the antibiotic, greatly increases the effectiveness of the latter without the need to increase the dosage.

Q: *Carrot juice is high in sugars. Does that not disturb the healing of diabetes?*

A: No. Carrot juice forms a very important part of healing. Rather than disturbing recovery, carrot juice provides the best source of vitamin A as well as most other vitamins. It is also one of the most complete sources of minerals containing most of the essential minerals in easily absorbed form. It is even high in vegetarian proteins and, for those reasons, it is an excellent source of total nutrition and healing.

Q: *With all the enemas being used in the course of the two years on the therapy, will I become dependent on enemas forever?*

A: No. Many patients, particularly women, have been constipated for some time, often for many years. When the liver and intestines are fully restored, most patients become "regular" again. Many of those who had been constipated recover "regularity." If not, it would be foolish to jeopardize recovery, when enemas are so important to heal and restore the body, just to be sure to remain "regular." In case the patient does lose their regularity, at worst they will have to take a daily enema as a morning routine. Dr. Gerson emphatically stressed, "Never let the sun set on a day when you haven't moved your bowel!"

Q: *On this therapy, without animal products, where do I get my proteins?*

A: As we have seen above, most vegetables contain adequate amounts of protein. This type of nutrient is easily absorbed, well digested and assimilated so that it produces healing—rather than feeding—tumor tissue, causing arthritic conditions, damaging kidneys, etc. The strongest and largest land animals (e.g., elephants, bulls and orangutans) are vegetarians and obtain their proteins from grass, plants, leaves and fruit. Carrot juice is high in proteins as are potatoes, oatmeal and most vegetables.

REFERENCES

1. M. Gerson, *A Cancer Therapy: Results of Fifty Cases and The Cure of Advanced Cancer by Diet Therapy: A Summary of Thirty Years of Clinical Experimentation,* 6th ed. (San Diego, CA: Gerson Institute, 1999), Appendix II, p. 418.
2. G. Matrone, et al., "Effect of Genistin on Growth and Development of the Male Mouse," *Journal of Nutrition* (1956): 235-240.
3. "Tomatoes, Tomato-Based Products, Lycopene, and Cancer: Review of the Epidemiologic Literature," *Journal of the National Cancer Institute* 91 (4) (Feb. 17, 1999): 317-331.
4. www.natural-cures-ear-sinus-infections.com/Antibiotic-Overuse.html
5. C. Woteki, J. Henney, *Strategy to Address the Problem of Agricultural Antimicrobial Use and the Emergence of Resistance.* FDA. Electronically published 10/2009; originally published 9/14/00 [cited 2010 0602]. Accessible at: www.fda.gov/downloads/animalveterinary/safetyhealth/antimicrobialresistance/UCM134773.pdf.

CHAPTER 26

Life After Gerson

C oming off the therapy at the right time has to be handled with care. Determining the right time is a tricky issue. To stop too soon, before all the essential organs are restored, is a great mistake, likely to lead to a recurrence. Patients suffering from nonmalignant diseases which respond well to the Gerson Therapy can be fully healed in a year or 18 months.

While coming off the treatment too soon is unwise, staying on it for "too long" does no harm. Stopping the therapy has to be a gradual process, slowly reducing the juices—if all goes well—reducing enemas to possibly two a week if the patient now has normal daily bowel movements and pain or headaches (symptoms of toxicity). Juices may be cut down to five or six a day, preferably indefinitely.

Eating Wisely

Changing over from the strict dietary rules to a more permissive regime also needs care. During the treatment, the body has gotten used to the best possible nutrition: fresh, pure, tasty, organic vegetarian food that is easily digested and provides all the necessary nutrients for health and fitness. It would be a grave mistake to switch from such a wholesome diet to the so-called normal variety—heavy with meat, poultry, cheese and chemically rich convenience foods—and risk a serious upset.

In our experience, recovered patients with their "clean" systems don't feel tempted by such foods even if, during the long treatment, they did fantasize about some "forbidden fruit." On the saltless Gerson regime, their taste buds have recovered from the paralysis caused by the highly salty foods of the past; now they find anything salty unpleasant and even offensive. (This is similar to former smokers who find it impossible to stay in a smoky room, let alone start smoking again.)

Of course, once a recovered patient is in a truly good condition with their systems working well, it is all right to attend a banquet, a wedding or a birthday celebration and "binge" a little. Afterwards, digestive enzymes should be taken for a few days, accompanied by a daily enema, to get rid of the mess and feel good again. **Please don't discard your enema bucket.** "Upside-down coffee," in Gerson parlance, helps if you have a headache, a toothache or even an incipient cold or a general malaise. Also, hang on to your Norwalk or other juicer instead of switching over to bottled juices; they won't help keep you well.

Patients who had been very seriously ill must take extra precautions to preserve their newfound health. **We suggest that, however long they have been off the therapy, they should go back on the full intensive program for two weeks, twice a year.** (Spring and fall, the times of seasonal changes, are best for this purpose.) During those two weeks, they should drink 10 to 13 juices a day, eat only freshly prepared organic foods, avoid animal proteins and take three or more enemas daily. If this return to the strict Gerson protocol produces a healing reaction, which these patients would recognize at once, the body is obviously clearing up some fresh damage and the strict program should be extended for another two weeks. If, however, no new symptoms pop up, the patient is doing well and can stop the "refresher course" after two weeks.

The Art of Maintenance

Originally, Dr. Gerson suggested that recovered patients should maintain their good health by ensuring that 75% of their diet consisted of "protective" foods—namely, organic fruits and vegetables high in nutrients, vitamins, minerals and enzymes—to keep the immune system in prime condition. The remaining 25% of food was to be "at choice." Unfortunately, this division is no longer applicable since the freely chosen foods would be far too damaging. We therefore have to urge former patients to stay with 90% of "protective" foods and have at most 10% of their intake consist of freely chosen items.

Even so, they should never return to fast foods, junk foods containing pesticides, food additives and other toxic stuff, and most certainly not items such as hot dogs, spiced meats and sausages laced with preservatives or cheese—the very foods that contributed to the breakdown of their health in the first place. However, if some serious dietary indiscretion occurs, it is wise to go back on the full therapy for a few weeks and clear up the body rather than risk long-term damage. **Obviously, great care must be taken with alcohol; very occasionally, a little wine may be enjoyed, but only if it is organic.** Commercially produced wines, made from frequently sprayed grapes, are to be avoided.

If you know what to avoid and what to hang on to, maintenance quickly becomes an easy and pleasant routine. **The answer to the question, "Is there life after Gerson?," is a clear and resounding yes!**

CHAPTER 27

Overcoming Stress and Tension

The Gerson program will also work best for the relaxed, unstressed patient. After all, it is not enough to eat the best possible food and drink the most health-giving juices; they also have to be digested and absorbed properly. It is no secret that anxiety and worry can wreak havoc with digestion.

Keeping mind and emotions on an even keel, banishing stress and fear must be part of the Gerson patient's daily routine. Fortunately, there are some simple, enjoyable methods that make this possible. In this chapter, we present a full range. Please try them and which suit you best.

Minding the Body

Posture can have a huge impact on how we feel, just as how we feel is often betrayed by our posture. When we are happy, we walk on air. When we are miserable, our head goes down, our shoulders move up and our back curves forward and slumps—all of which compress our innards and add to the gloom. That will never do.

Learn to keep your spine straight but not rigid, both standing and sitting. (Please freeze for a moment and check what your spine is doing.)

Sit with both feet on the ground and don't cross your legs; doing so impedes the circulation and twists the spine. Walk from the hips and avoid leaning forward, as if you were pushing a grocery cart. You can't get ahead of yourself! Think of your head as the hook of a coat hanger, with your body hanging from it loosely and comfortably. The shoulders are a particularly tension-prone part of the body. They tend to move forward and up, whenever we feel stressed, as if wanting to protect the chest. A side effect of this unconscious move is that anxious people seem to have short necks. In the memorable words of a yoga teacher, opening up your chest means saying yes to life.

Make sure your shoulders are where they belong. Stand up straight, draw both shoulders up as far as they will go, right up to the earlobes, and then drop them as if they had become redundant. Where they land is their natural position. Please memorize it for future use.

It is also helpful to keep your neck supple and relaxed (and make it longer!) by regular exercise. Turn your head slowly from left to right and back. Drop your head gently forward and backward, keeping your lower jaw loose. Rotate your head first clockwise, then counterclockwise, repeating each movement five times. If at any time you feel you are tensing up, imagine that you are a rag doll in a strong breeze and move accordingly.

Hands are also tension-prone. They tend to curl into fists as soon as we feel anxious or angry. In old Western films, you could tell that things were getting dangerous when the hero's knuckles turned white. Actually, anybody's knuckles can turn white from fear and this is what needs to be avoided. Train yourself to keep your fingers splayed when your hands are at rest. That prevents the tensing up of the arms, which would lead to further tension rushing through the body. If at first you fail and all you have are fists, imagine that you have washed your hands and have no towel, so that you need to shake both hands vigorously from the wrists. As you do that, feel the tension dropping away from your fingertips.

Breathing deserves our full attention. Breath is the basic condition of life. We can live for quite a while without food and for a much shorter time without water, but life without breath ends in a few moments.

Most of us neglect this vital function until we learn otherwise and switch from shallow to deep abdominal breathing. This way, routinely used by singers, speakers, practitioners of yoga and athletes, boosts the body's oxygen intake and has a calming effect.

The method is simplicity itself. With each in-breath, push out your stomach so that the breath can fill your lungs to full capacity. Fill your lower lungs first, then the middle of your lungs and finally your upper lungs. Hold your breath for a second or two and then, as you breathe out, pull in your stomach hard, squeezing out the stale air. Find your own rhythm and practice this method several times a day until it becomes your natural way of breathing. If at first it is a bit difficult, imagine that, in your abdomen, there is a beautiful balloon, which you inflate with each in-breath and deflate by letting the air out. You will be surprised what a difference better breathing makes to your well-being.

Matters of the Mind

Your mental attitude can be your best ally—or your worst enemy— and the same applies to your imagination, depending on how you use it. Positively used, your thoughts and ideas can help you to reprogram your entire outlook, your moods and your feelings so that they promote health and healing instead of dragging you down. Energy follows thought!

There are several ways to achieve the best possible state of mind. All of them depend on your ability to relax as fully as possible so that no tension interferes with what you are trying to do. The simplest way is to lie on your back on a comfortable but not too soft surface, with your hands loosely resting by your sides. Close your eyes. Start breathing slowly, deeply, from the abdomen. With each in-breath, imagine drawing in brilliant light, which fills you with peace, strength and energy. With each out-breath, imagine releasing all tiredness, tension, pain or anxiety in the shape of dirty, dark smoke. Let your head and your body become very heavy so that the floor carries your weight. Check through your body, starting with your toes and working your way up to the top of your head, for traces of tension or stiffness, and release them.

Make sure your jaw is relaxed and your tongue lies easy against your upper palate. Stay with this feeling of peace, release and relaxation for a little while.

This basic letting-go is the key to all kinds of inner work, including meditation, prayer, visualization and affirmations. Practiced at least twice a day, free from disturbance, noise and interruptions, it will make a great difference to your mental state, which in turn will affect your body.

Meditation

Meditation is a simple way to still the ever-busy brain and enter a place of profound stillness and peace which, for a short while, lets us escape from everyday reality. It needs practice; the brain is hard to discipline and keeps bringing in thoughts, fragments of ideas and all kinds of mental rubbish. At first, you may find that even 30 seconds of stillness is quite an achievement. Don't give up! There are ways to improve the situation.

One way is to get hold of intruding thoughts, identify them, imagine tying a big balloon to each one and watch them float away. Another way is to improve concentration by counting from one to four, seeing in your mind's eye the numbers, shining bright and beautiful against 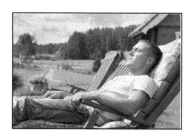 a dark curtain, and repeat the counting 10 times. You can also place a clock at eye level and fix your entire attention to the second hand going round and round so that nothing else matters. Gradually—but with perseverance—you'll find it easier to achieve spells of thought-free awareness, leading to an extraordinary sense of restfulness and peace.

Switching off the brain for a little while also enables us to hear our so-called inner voice—the voice of intuition and wisdom. Whatever our belief system, and whether or not we are religious, we all have an inner life and a set of values by which we live. Often, it is at a time of crisis, caused by a serious health breakdown, that we turn inward and review our position in life. Naturally, Gerson patients are totally free to choose their own way in this field; we are all different and must respect our differences. However, it is the experience of many doctors, counselors and other health professionals that patients who believe in a higher reality, who are able to pray and put their faith in God, fare better than those who don't. Prayer, coming from the heart, with trust in the ultimate rightness of things, can be a great support on the rocky path of recovery.

Visualization

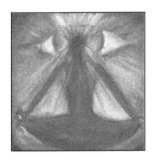

Visualization uses the imagination to reprogram not only the mind but, to a certain extent, the body. It works through images, bypassing the thinking-talking brain, and those images come from the same deep area of the psyche as the ones we meet in our dreams. The purpose of visualization is to prescribe, so to speak, what we want to achieve: defeating disease, rebuilding health, recovering and living a full life. Using visualization in the context of cancer was first developed in the 1970s by the American radiation oncologist Carl Simonton, MD. *Getting Well Again,*[1] the book he wrote with his then-wife, psychologist Stephanie Matthews-Simonton, has appeared in many editions and several languages.

The essence of the Simonton technique is to find one image for the disease and another one for the treatment, and how the latter attacks and gradually demolishes the former. For instance, in the state of deep relaxation described above, the Gerson patient may visualize his or her tumor as a big blob of black mud, and the juices as powerful bursts of golden liquid that attack and gradually clear away the mud. Read cold from the page, this may sound odd; practiced as it is meant to be, it can be a powerful experience.

Here is a simple visualization exercise for daily use: yourself in a perfectly beautiful place, real or imaginary, where you feel safe, secure and happy. Make yourself comfortable in imagination, in whatever way feels right for you: gently swaying in a soft hammock, walking in a perfect garden or sitting happily with a loved one. Choose your own setting outside time and space and be refreshed by its peace and beauty.

Now yourself as you wish to be: healthy, fit, strong and active, doing the things you most enjoy, able to give and receive love and feeling at home in the world. Surrender to this image, become it and anchor it in your mind and heart, then slowly return to mundane reality but bring with you the memory of the experience. It does make a difference. Actually, a similar technique is used by successful sportsmen and sportswomen who, before an important event, visualize themselves doing extremely well in their chosen area.

Imagination is powerful. Used well, it stimulates and tunes the body. It is free, nontoxic and has no harmful side effects, which makes it the ideal supplementary tool for Gerson patients.

REFERENCE

1. Carl Simonton, MD, James L. Creighton and Stephanie Matthews-Simonton, *Getting Well Again* (New York: Bantam Books, reissue edition April 1, 1992).

CHAPTER 28

Recipes

L ast, but far from least, this chapter contains a treasury of recipes that add variety, pleasure and super-healthy nutrition to Gerson-style meals. However, there are some important points to remember:

- Study and learn by heart the basic rules for food preparation described in Chapter 17, "Preparing Food and Juices —The Basic Rules," p. 147.

- If you are a Gerson patient, newly embarked on the full therapy, you need to limit your food intake to the basic recipes contained in that chapter for the first three months and eat no dairy products for the first six to 10 weeks.

- After three months, you may introduce some variety by using different salads, dressings and vegetable courses.

- The "Special Soup or Hippocrates Soup" and the baked potato are essential parts of the healing diet and must not be omitted.

If you are not ill but wish to improve your health and well-being by switching to the Gerson lifestyle, you may of course enjoy the recipes freely. Please use the slow, low heat, waterless or minimum-water cooking method, described in Chapter 12, in order to preserve precious nutrients.

Patients diagnosed with collagen diseases should avoid citrus fruit and orange or grapefruit juices. Use freshly pressed apple juice or apple/carrot juice in their place.

Special Notes

Bread

You will find no recipes for bread or other flour-based baked goods in this chapter. The only acceptable bread—unsalted, organic 100% rye bread—is available at good health food stores, so there is no point in baking bread at home. Patients are allowed two small slices of bread a day, but only after eating the complete Gerson meals consisting of salad, soup and potato with vegetables and fruit. Bread must not take the place of any of these items.

Yogurt

Yogurt, when permitted, must be certified organic and fat free (or extremely low fat). A few recipes refer to "yogurt." To make this, hang some regular yogurt, placed in several layers of cheesecloth, over the sink or in a cheesecloth-lined strainer over a bowl, and allow it to drain overnight

Sweeteners

The only permitted sweeteners are:

- Organic raw brown sugar, which is available in various shades ranging from light beige to dark brown

- Organic clear honey

- Organic maple syrup

- Unsulphured molasses

- Sucanat (also known as rapadura)

In the recipes, these ingredients are referred to as "honey" and "sugar."

Washing Fruits and Vegetables

All fruits and vegetables must be washed before use. If the water supply in your area is not fluoridated, purified water (produced by reverse osmosis) may be used, both for washing produce and for cooking. If the water supply contains fluoride, only distilled water is permissible for cooking and as a final rinse for fruits and vegetables. (For distillers, see Chapter 14, "The Gerson Household," p. 128.)

Baking

When baking, the oven should always be preheated.

Cooking Time/Serving Size

When a specific cooking time or a number of people served is omitted, it is because it depends on the size of the ingredients. For example, if a large potato is used, it takes much more time to bake or cook than a small one. Also, one or two large potatoes serve more people than the same number of small ones.

Special Soup or Hippocrates Soup

"Special Soup" or "Hippocrates Soup" are interchangeable terms for the same staple item of the Gerson diet. In some recipes, it is referred to as "soup stock." For a detailed description, see Chapter 17, "Preparing Food and Juices —The Basic Rules," p. 147.

Bon appetit!

Recipes

Dips

Carrot and Dill Dip

Preparation time: 15 minutes
Cooking time: 30 minutes
Serves 4-8

1 lb. carrots, scrubbed, unpeeled
4 tbsp. yogurt
2 tbsp. dill weed (or 2 tsp. dried dill), finely chopped
1 tsp. flaxseed oil
juice of 1 small lemon

Simmer carrots until just tender. Drain and leave until cooled. Put through the food mill. Mix in yogurt, dill, flaxseed oil and lemon juice. Mix well. Chill in the refrigerator. Serve as part of a large salad or as a dip with carrot, zucchini and bell pepper sticks. Also delicious on bread.

Orange (or Red) Pepper Dip

Preparation time: 15 minutes
Serves 6

2 orange (or red) bell peppers

10 oz. yogurt

1/2 tsp. organic tomato purée

Seed and dice one of the peppers very finely and mix with the yogurt and tomato purée. Slice the remaining pepper lengthwise in half and remove the seeds. Place the yogurt mixture into each pepper half. Place on a serving dish with thin strips of carrot, zucchini and celery.

Appetizers

Celery Root Rémoulade Appetizer

Preparation Time: 10 minutes
Serves 2-4

celery root
radicchio lettuce
2 or 3 varieties of loose leaf lettuce (butter or red leaf lettuce)
green onions (or chives), chopped
parsley (or tarragon)

Dressing:
vinegar
water
honey
yogurt

Combine the dressing ingredients. Grate the celery root and add the dressing. Place lettuce leaves on a plate and top with celery root. Sprinkle with chopped green onions (or chives) and parsley (or tarragon).

Eggplant Appetizer

Preparation time: 15 minutes
Cooking time: 50 minutes
Serves 2

1 eggplant
1 small onion, chopped
1/2 tbsp. organic tomato purée
parsley (or cilantro)
lemon wedge
yogurt

Prick the skin of the eggplant all over. Place directly onto the oven rack (or use a small baking dish) and bake at 375° F (190° C) for about 40 minutes near the top of the oven, turning once after 20 minutes.

Remove from oven and cool. When cool, peel away the stalk and skin, and chop the flesh until you have a rough purée. Heat a little water in a small pan and sauté the chopped onion over low heat for about 10 minutes or until soft. Stir in the tomato purée and the eggplant purée. Cook for another 2 minutes over high heat to remove excess moisture. Remove from heat and cool completely. Chop some parsley (or cilantro) and mix in with the purée. Lay on a bed of lettuce. Garnish with a wedge of lemon and a little yogurt.

Grapefruit Appetizer

Preparation time: 15 minutes
Serves 1 or 2

1 pink grapefruit
celery
1 red bell pepper, seeded
radicchio (or red leaf lettuce leaves)
grated horseradish

Cut the grapefruit in half. Juice one-half and cut out the segments of the other half. Chop some celery and seeded red pepper. Arrange a layer of radicchio (or red leaf lettuce leaves) on a plate. Mix grapefruit segments, celery and red pepper together and put on top of lettuce. Make a dressing with grapefruit juice flavored with a little grated horseradish (or chopped mint leaves).

Variation: Put grapefruit segments on top of endive and watercress. Make a dressing with yogurt and a little grapefruit juice. Mix well and serve immediately.

How to segment a grapefruit: Cut a horizontal slice off the top and bottom. Sit the grapefruit flat and, using a sharp knife, remove the peel and outer white membrane by cutting downwards in sections. Using a container to catch any juice, cut between the membranes and the flesh of each segment to the core, taking care to point the knife blade away from you. Work around the grapefruit, easing out each segment as you go.

Jerusalem Artichoke Paté

Preparation time: 20 minutes
Cooking time: 40 minutes
Serves 2

1 lb. Jerusalem artichokes
1 tbsp. yogurt
1-2 tsp. lemon juice
parsley, chopped
flaxseed oil

Scrub the artichokes. Put in dish in oven to roast at 400° F (204° C) for 25 minutes. (It's a good idea to cook them with your baked potato.) Allow to cool and remove skin. Mash or purée (with electric blender or food mill) until it has a creamy consistency. Add the yogurt, lemon juice, chopped parsley and flaxseed oil, and beat together. Serve as an appetizer or a snack with toasted slices of bread and a smattering of various lettuce leaves and cherry tomatoes to decorate.

Melon and Mango Appetizer

Preparation time: 15 minutes
Serves 2-4

slices of honeydew and/or cantaloupe melon
slices of mango

Dressing:
1/2 tbsp. honey
1 tbsp. flaxseed oil
2 tbsp. lime (or lemon) juice
mint leaves

Cut the melon in half and remove the rind. Slice the melon and arrange in a fan shape on a shallow plate. Slice the mango lengthwise and peel, including the flesh left around the pit. Cut the mango flesh into slices and arrange between the melon slices on the plate. Pour the dressing over the melon.

Papaya and Lime Appetizer

Preparation time: 15 minutes
Serves 2

2 papayas
2 tbsp. honey
juice of 1 lime
1 lime for decoration, sliced

Peel the papaya and remove the seeds. Cut into slices (or cubes). Mix the honey with the lime juice and pour over papaya slices. Toss gently and refrigerate. Serve chilled, decorated with thin slices of lime.

Stuffed Zucchini Appetizer

Preparation time: 10 minutes
Cooking time: 5 minutes
Serves 2-4

8 medium zucchinis
1 large onion, chopped
1 green bell pepper
3 tomatoes
1 tsp. parsley, chopped
1 clove garlic, crushed
red leaf lettuce
4-6 tbsp. dressing

Dressing:
6 tbsp. apple cider vinegar (or lemon juice)
4 tbsp. water
herbs
flaxseed oil

Cook the zucchini whole (about 5 minutes on a very low heat) until half-cooked. Cut off both ends and cut each in half lengthwise. Scoop out the seeds and chop them. Sprinkle some dressing into the zucchini hollows and add a little chopped onion. Leave to marinate while preparing the stuffing. Take the remaining onion and chop the pepper and tomatoes, add the chopped parsley and crushed garlic, and mix with the chopped zucchini middles. Toss in the rest of the dressing and fill the hollows with the mixture. Arrange on a layer of red leaf lettuce to serve.

Yogurt and Apricot Sorbet Appetizer

Freezing time: 2-3 hours
Preparation time: 15 minutes
Cooking time: 40 minutes
Serves 2-4

8 oz. dried apricots
20 fl. oz. water
10 oz. yogurt
2 tbsp. honey

Place the apricots and a little water in a saucepan and bring to a boil. Cover and simmer for 30-40 minutes, or until soft. Add the rest of the water to bring the liquid content to 15 oz. Leave to cool. Place the apricots and liquid in a blender and blend until smooth. Add the yogurt and honey but do not blend these. Transfer the contents to a freeze-proof container and freeze until solid. Use an ice-cream scooper to serve one or two scoops into a bowl. Serve immediately.

Dressings

Baba Ghanoush (Eggplant and Lemon Dressing)

Preparation time: 10 minutes
Cooking time: 1 hour
Serves 3 or 4

1 large eggplant
1 or 2 cloves garlic
2 tbsp. lemon juice
1 tbsp. parsley, chopped

Bake the eggplant for 1 hour at 350-400° F (177-204° C). When cooled enough to peel, drain off excess juice, squeezing gently. Mash and blend with garlic until fairly smooth and add lemon juice and parsley. Mix well. Serve with lemon wedges. Good with crudités (raw veggies) and as a relish as well as a sauce.

Variation: Mix with yogurt.

Basic Salad Dressing

Preparation time: 7 minutes
Serves 2

2 tbsp. lemon juice (or apple cider vinegar)
2 tbsp. water
pinch of sugar (optional)

Mix together and put into a container with any of the following:
tarragon, pushed in stalk first
shallots (or green onions), finely chopped
2 cloves garlic, peeled and crushed
fresh bay leaf
lemon grass (for a lemon flavor)

Dressing for Vegetables

Preparation time: 5 minutes
Serves 2

2 tbsp. lemon juice (or apple cider vinegar)
2 tbsp. water
pinch of sugar (optional)
yogurt

Mix lemon juice (or apple cider vinegar), water and sugar (if used). Mix in yogurt and beat well.

Flaxseed Oil and Lemon Juice Dressing

Preparation time: 5 minutes
Serves 2

1 tbsp. flaxseed oil
1/2 tbsp. lemon juice
(Use a ratio of 2/3 oil to 1/3 lemon juice)
garlic
fresh herbs
a little orange juice

Combine all the ingredients in a pitcher and stir vigorously. Pour over the salad and serve immediately.

Garlic and Green Onion Dressing

Preparation time: 5 minutes
Serves 1

1 tbsp. flaxseed oil
1/2 tbsp. lemon juice (or apple cider vinegar)
1 clove garlic
1 green onion
fresh parsley
chives
dill
fennel
a little mint

Mix flaxseed oil with lemon juice (or apple cider vinegar). Crush the garlic and add. Chop the green onion, parsley and chives and add, together with the dill, fennel and mint. Either pour over the salad and serve immediately, or put into a pitcher and allow guests to serve themselves.

Variation: If you have no fresh herbs, use a generous pinch of suitable dried herbs.

Basic Dressing

Preparation time: 5 minutes
Serves 6

2-1/3 cup apple cider vinegar
1 tsp. sugar
2/3 cup water

Mix ingredients together.

Variation: Add some or all of the following herbs (optional), letting them infuse: tarragon (pushed in stalk first); shallots or spring onions, finely chopped; 2 cloves of garlic, peeled and crushed with the back of a knife; and 1 fresh bay leaf.

Orange Vinaigrette

Preparation time: 6 minutes
Serves 1

1 clove garlic
2 tbsp. fresh parsley
2 tbsp. apple cider vinegar
1 tsp. sugar
4 tbsp. orange juice
1 tbsp. flaxseed oil

Chop the garlic and parsley, and add to vinegar, sugar, orange juice and flaxseed oil.

Yogurt, Garlic and Honey Dressing

Preparation time: 6 minutes
Serves 2

6 oz. yogurt
1 clove garlic, crushed
1 tsp. honey
watercress

Mix the ingredients, toss lightly and serve immediately. Garnish with watercress.

Yogurt, Herb and Vinegar Dressing

Preparation time: 4 minutes

apple cider vinegar
a little water
honey
yogurt
parsley
tarragon

Mix all together.

Yogurt, Onion and Apple Cider Vinegar Dressing

Preparation time: 4 minutes

yogurt
apple cider vinegar
chopped onion

Mix all together and serve with a green salad.

Salads

Apple and Carrot Salad

Preparation time: 15 minutes
Serves 2

1 small crisp red apple
1 large carrot
1 green onion, chopped
1 radish, sliced
apple juice
mint

Grate the apple and carrot into a dish and add a chopped green onion and a sliced radish. Pour over a little apple juice and sprinkle with mint. Serve on a bed of mixed colored salad leaves, such as radicchio, watercress or parsley.

Beet and Watercress Salad

Preparation time: 5 minutes

cooked beet
flaxseed oil
watercress

Chop cooked beet and toss in a little flaxseed oil. Serve with watercress.

Beet Salad Yolande

Preparation time: 20 minutes

cooked beets
carrots
celery
apples
parsley

Dressing:
yogurt
lemon juice
flaxseed oil

Dice the beets, carrots, celery and apples and put into a bowl. Make the dressing and mix in with the vegetables. Sprinkle with parsley.

Beet Thermidor

Preparation time: 6 minutes

cooked beets

Dressing:
yogurt

lemon juice
grated horseradish

Dice cooked beets, put into a bowl and add the dressing.

Carrot Salad

Preparation time: 15 minutes
Serves 2-4

8 oz. carrots
1 medium crisp eating apple
5 oz. yogurt
juice of 1 large orange

Grate the carrots into a bowl. Cut the apple into quarters, remove core, then grate into the bowl and mix with the carrot. Mix the yogurt with the orange juice and stir into the salad.

Variation: Presoaked raisins (soak overnight in cold water, or pour boiling water over them and leave for a couple of hours until plump) or sultanas can also be added.

Carrot and Orange Salad with Fresh Dates

Preparation time: 15 minutes
Serves 2

1 large carrot
1 orange
a few fresh dates
toasted oats

Dressing:
lemon (or lime) juice
flaxseed oil

Cut the carrot into thin strips. Segment the orange and mix with the carrot. Chop the dates and add. Add dressing and garnish with toasted oats.

Carrot and Raisin Salad

Preparation time: 10 minutes*
* Does not include presoaking
Serves 2

3 large carrots, grated
2 oz. raisins, presoaked
lettuce
2 tsp. parsley, chopped

Dressing:
1 clove garlic, crushed
flaxseed oil
apple cider vinegar
1/2 tsp. honey
2 tsp. lemon juice

Mix grated raw carrots with presoaked raisins (soak the raisins overnight in cold water, or pour boiling water over them and leave for a couple of hours until plump). Add dressing and serve on lettuce garnished with chopped parsley.

Carrot, Apple and Onion Salad

Preparation time: 15 minutes
Serves 2

12 oz. carrots
8 oz. apples
1 medium onion
10 oz. yogurt
juice of 1/2 lemon

Shred the carrots, apples and onion. Combine with the yogurt and lemon juice. Serve with a mixed green salad.

Celery Salad

Preparation time: 10 minutes
Serves 2

2 stalks celery
2 crisp small eating apples
1/4 medium red bell pepper, finely sliced
mixed lettuce leaves

Dressing:
apple cider vinegar
flaxseed oil
1 tsp. honey

Chop the celery and apples and put into a large bowl. Add the finely sliced red bell pepper. Add the dressing. Line a salad plate with mixed lettuce leaves and pile the dressed salad on top.

Cherry Tomato and Watercress Relish

Preparation time: 15 minutes
Serves 2-4

cherry tomatoes (red and yellow)
watercress
fresh chives (or green onions), finely chopped
herbs, finely chopped

Halve the tomatoes and place in a bowl. Steam the watercress over boiling water for 10 seconds, rinse well in cold water and shake dry. Trim off any woody stems and cut or tear the remaining stems and leaves into small pieces. Add to the tomatoes. Add the finely chopped chives (or green onions) and herbs and toss together.

Chicory and Orange Salad

Preparation time: 15 minutes
Serves 2-4

1 lb. chicory heads

2 large oranges
1 medium green onion
juice of 1/2 lemon
1 tbsp. flaxseed oil
1 tsp. honey

Trim the chicory and slice into rounds about 1/2-inch thick. Push the rounds apart to make rings. Peel the oranges, removing the white pith, and slice into rounds. Place the chicory in a bowl and lay the oranges in overlapping rings around the top, leaving the center empty. Trim and chop the green onion and sprinkle into the center. Mix the lemon juice, flaxseed oil and honey, and pour over the salad. Leave for a few minutes before serving to allow the flavors to "marry."

Coleslaw

Preparation time: 15 minutes*
* Does not include presoaking

raisins
white cabbage
apple
celery
onion

Dressing:
yogurt
lemon juice
flaxseed oil

Presoak the raisins (soak the raisins overnight in cold water, or pour boiling water over them and leave for a couple of hours until plump). Thinly shred the white cabbage and apple. Finely chop the celery and onion. Put all into a bowl and add the raisins. Toss in dressing.

Colorful Mixed Salad

Preparation time: 15 minutes
Serves 2

zucchini
beet
apple
lettuce
tomato
orange

Dressing:
equal amounts of apple cider vinegar and water
honey (or maple syrup)
garlic
lemon (or orange) juice

Grate the zucchini, beet and apple. Add the dressing and mix them together or pile them in separate mounds onto a bed of lettuce. Decorate with slices of tomatoes and orange.

Colorful Three-Cabbage Salad

Preparation time: 15 minutes*
* Does not include presoaking
Serves 2

2 oz. raisins
4 oz. each white, red and green cabbage
4 oz. carrot
1 medium onion, finely sliced
1 small crisp eating apple, chopped
watercress

Dressing:
5 fl. oz. yogurt
a little flaxseed oil
1 clove garlic, crushed

Presoak the raisins (soak the raisins overnight in cold water, or pour boiling water over them and leave for a couple of hours until plump). Finely shred the cabbage. Grate the carrot. Put both in a bowl with the raisins, finely sliced onion and chopped apple. Mix well. Mix the dressing ingredients and pour over the salad just before serving, tossing lightly. Garnish with watercress.

Colorful Winter Salad

Preparation time: 20 minutes
Serves 4-6

3 tart eating apples
lemon juice
1/4 medium-sized red cabbage
1 medium carrot
1/2 medium red bell pepper
2 sticks celery
1/2 red onion
watercress

Core and roughly chop the apples and mix with lemon juice in a small bowl. Core and finely shred the red cabbage. Peel and grate the carrot. (This is the only time to peel the carrots. If they are grated with their skins on, they tend to turn brown.) Seed and chop the red pepper. Slice the celery. Peel and chop the red onion. Put all the above ingredients into a large bowl. Garnish with watercress.

Variations: Serve with cottage cheese (unsalted and uncreamed or fat-free) and your favorite dressing.

Crunchy Salad

Preparation time: 15 minutes*
* Does not include presoaking
Serves 4-6

2 oz. dried apricots, chopped
3 oz. raisins

1 lb. white cabbage
1 green bell pepper
1 red bell pepper (or 1/2 bunch of radishes)
watercress

Dressing:
6 fl. oz. yogurt
1 clove garlic, crushed
1 tsp. honey

Presoak the apricots and raisins (soak overnight in cold water, or pour boiling water over them and leave for a couple of hours until plump). Finely shred the white cabbage. Chop the pepper (or radishes). Place into a bowl together with the raisins and chopped apricots. Mix well. Mix the dressing and pour over the salad. Toss lightly, garnish with watercress and serve.

Endive and Orange Salad

Preparation time: 15 minutes
Serves 2

1 small head of endive
1 red bell pepper
2 oranges
2 tomatoes
1 tbsp. herbs, chopped

Dressing:
juice of 2 oranges
5 oz. yogurt
1 tsp. honey

Chop the endive and put into a bowl. Seed the pepper, cut into thin strips and add to the bowl. Peel the oranges, removing the pith with the peel. Cut out segments between the membranes and add to the bowl with the tomatoes. Make the dressing and toss into the salad. Sprinkle with chopped herbs.

Fruity Winter Salad

Preparation time: 15 minutes*
* Does not include presoaking
Serves 2-4

2 oz. raisins
2 oz. dried figs
2 oz. dried apricots
1/2 white cabbage
2 carrots
2 red eating apples
8 tbsp. yogurt
1 lemon
parsley, chopped

Presoak the raisins, figs and apricots (soak overnight in cold water, or pour boiling water over them and leave for a couple of hours until plump). Finely shred the cabbage. Coarsely grate the carrots and apples. (Sprinkle the apples with lemon juice to stop them from turning brown.) Put the above ingredients into a bowl. Combine the yogurt, lemon juice and chopped parsley in a jug and spoon over the salad. Toss together until well mixed.

Gerson Coleslaw

Preparation time: 15 minutes
Serves 2-4

onion
white cabbage
carrot

Dressing:
2 tbsp. lemon juice
2 tbsp. water
sugar (optional)
yogurt
cottage cheese (unsalted and uncreamed or fat-free)

Slice or chop the onion. Grate or slice the white cabbage. Grate the carrot. Mix all together. For the dressing, mix lemon juice with water (and sugar, if used). Mix yogurt with cottage cheese and beat well to get rid of any lumps. Then add the lemon juice and water mixture. Mix well and pour over salad.

Grated Zucchini Salad with Lime

Preparation time: 15 minutes
Serves 2-4

1 lb. zucchini
juice of 1 lime (or lemon)
1 red bell pepper, grated
1 clove garlic, crushed
lettuce

Grate the zucchini finely. Mix with the lime (or lemon) juice and grated pepper. Add crushed garlic. Allow the flavors to blend a little before serving on a bed of lettuce.

Hungarian Tomato Salad

Preparation time: 15 minutes

whole tomatoes
lettuce
chopped chives

Dressing:
yogurt
lemon juice
flaxseed oil
grated horseradish

Skin the tomatoes by dipping them in boiling water for a minute. Make the dressing. Place the whole, skinned tomatoes on the lettuce leaves and cover with the dressing. Garnish with chopped chives.

Jumbo Salad

Preparation time: 20 minutes
Does not include presoaking
Serves 4-6

variety of shredded lettuce leaves
and salad greens, bite-sized and shredded

Any, or all, of the following:
tomato, chopped
green (or red) bell pepper, chopped
green onions, finely sliced
carrot
beet
radish, finely sliced
fennel, finely sliced
grape halves
lemon juice
flaxseed oil
dried dill weed
raisins, presoaked

Gradually build up the salad, beginning with the bite-sized shredded lettuce leaves and salad greens. Add any, or all, of the ingredients listed above. Presoak the raisins (soak overnight in cold water, or pour boiling water over them and leave for a couple of hours until plump). Sprinkle on top of the salad. Grate the carrot and/or beet and place to one side of the salad. (If you put it all on top, it tends to "smother" the salad.) Pour on the lemon juice and flaxseed oil. Sprinkle with dill. Serve with rice, oven-cooked and sliced potatoes or boiled small new potatoes.

Minted Apple and Celery Salad

Preparation time: 15 minutes
* *Does not include presoaking*
Serves 2

1 red eating apple

apple cider vinegar
1 stalk of celery
raisins, presoaked
mint leaves
lettuce

Cut and core the apple and chop into bite-sized chunks. Mix with a little apple cider vinegar (diluted with water, if desired). Chop the celery and add, with the presoaked raisins (soak overnight in cold water, or pour boiling water over them and leave for a couple of hours until plump), to the apple and apple cider vinegar. Take the mint leaves and tear into small pieces. Add to the dish and serve on a bed of lettuce. (Leave for a little while before serving so the flavors have time to mix.)

Variation: Yogurt can be mixed with the apple cider vinegar for the dressing.

Orange, Chicory and Watercress Salad

Preparation time: 15 minutes
Serves 2-4

1 orange
2 heads of chicory
1 bunch of watercress

Dressing:
1 tbsp. flaxseed oil
1/2 tbsp. apple cider vinegar (or lemon juice)
1 clove garlic, crushed
1 green onion
parsley
chives
dill
fennel
mint

Peel the orange and split into segments. Separate the chicory leaves and arrange like the spokes of a wheel around a large dish. Put the watercress and orange in the middle. Combine all the dressing ingredients in a jug and stir vigorously. (If you have no fresh herbs, use a generous pinch of dried herbs.) Pour over the salad and serve immediately.

Radish, Apple and Celery Salad

Preparation time: 15 minutes*
* Does not include presoaking
Serves 2

radishes
green apples
celery
raisins
lettuce

Dressing:
1 tbsp. apple cider vinegar
1 tbsp. water
1 tsp. sugar (or honey)
1 or 2 cloves garlic, crushed
dill, chopped
yogurt

Chop the radishes, green apples and celery into small chunks. Presoak the raisins (soak overnight in cold water, or pour boiling water over them and leave for a couple of hours until plump) and add. For the dressing, mix together the apple cider vinegar, water, sugar (or honey), garlic and dill. Add enough yogurt to make a creamy dressing. Pour over the salad and serve on a bed of lettuce (include radicchio or red leaf, if available).

Variations: Use other herbs instead of dill, omit the yogurt or add some flaxseed oil.

Raw Turnip, Watercress and Orange Salad

Preparation time: 15 minutes
Serves 2

1 turnip
1 orange
watercress

Dressing:
orange juice
flaxseed oil

Peel and cut the turnip into matchstick-size pieces. Segment the orange and add to the turnip pieces. Add the watercress and toss in the dressing.

Rice Salad

Preparation time: 15 minutes
Serves 2

green bell pepper
red bell pepper
tomato
1 cup cooked brown rice

Dressing:
1 tbsp. flaxseed oil
1 tbsp. apple cider vinegar
1 clove garlic
sugar

Chop the peppers and tomato. Prepare the dressing, mix well and add the chopped peppers and tomato. Spoon onto the rice. Serve with a mixed green salad.

Romaine Lettuce with Yogurt Dressing

Preparation time: 10 minutes

Romaine lettuce
chives, chopped

Dressing:
yogurt
sugar
lemon juice
crushed garlic

Coarsely shred the lettuce. Pour on the dressing and sprinkle with chopped chives.

Salad Kebabs

Preparation time: 15 minutes

tomatoes
zucchinis
whole radishes
lettuce hearts
carrots

Dressing:
lemon juice
yogurt
flaxseed oil
herbs (mint, dill or parsley)

Thread on wooden skewers thinly sliced pieces of tomato, zucchini, whole radishes, lettuce hearts and raw carrot. Dip into the salad dressing before serving.

Salad Lorette

Preparation time: 10 minutes

cooked beets

celery stalks
lettuce

Dressing:
flaxseed oil
lemon juice

Thinly slice the beets and celery and mix with lettuce. Add dressing.

Spanish Salad

Preparation time: 15 minutes
Serves 2

onions
1 clove garlic
red bell peppers
tomatoes, sliced
parsley, chopped

Dressing:
flaxseed oil
1 tbsp. apple cider vinegar
1 tbsp. water
sugar (optional)

Thinly slice the onions and put into a bowl which has been rubbed over with a cut clove of garlic. Seed and slice the red peppers and lay them on top of the onion. Add a layer of sliced tomatoes. Crush the garlic and sprinkle on top. Pour over the dressing and sprinkle with chopped parsley.

Tomato and Zucchini Salad

Preparation time: 15 minutes
Serves 2

tomato
zucchini
green onion

beet
lettuce

Dressing:
flaxseed oil
yogurt
lemon juice

Chop the tomato and zucchini into chunks. Slice the green onion and add. Finely grate the raw beet (or chop cooked beet into chunks) and mix into the salad. Lay on a bed of lettuce. Pour over dressing.

Tomato Salad

Preparation time: 15 minutes
Serves 2

tomatoes
onion
1 tbsp. apple cider vinegar
1 tbsp. water
sugar (optional)
parsley, chopped
chives

Slice the tomatoes and spread out over a flat dish. Slice the onion and arrange the onion rings over the tomatoes. Mix the apple cider vinegar with water (and optional sugar, if used). Pour over the tomatoes and sprinkle with chopped parsley and chives.

Watercress, Endive and Grapefruit Salad

Preparation time: 10 minutes
Serves 2

watercress
endive (frisée or escarole, or both)
grapefruit
yogurt

Tear the watercress into smaller pieces, remove woody stems and put in a bowl with the endive leaves. Cut the grapefruit in half. Juice one half and segment the other half. Add the segments to salad leaves. Mix the grapefruit juice with yogurt and pour over the salad. Toss well and serve.

Zucchini Ribbon Salad

Preparation time: 10 minutes
Serves 2-4

3 large zucchinis
1 lb. tomatoes
6 green onions

Dressing:
2 tbsp. apple cider vinegar
pinch of sugar
2 tbsp. flaxseed oil
freshly chopped cilantro

Using a vegetable peeler or cheese slicer, cut the zucchinis lengthwise into thin ribbons, running along the side so the ribbons include the green skin. Place into a bowl. Quarter the tomatoes and thinly slice the onions. Add to the bowl. Toss in the dressing just before serving.

Soups

Apple and Fennel Soup

Preparation time: 15 minutes
Cooking time: 30-45 minutes
Serves 4

1 lb. potatoes
2 bulbs fennel
2 leeks
2 Granny Smith apples
1 tsp. sugar (optional)

1 tart eating apple

Peel and dice the potatoes, trim and chop the fennel, slice the leeks, and core and chop the apples into small pieces. Put these ingredients into a pot and cover with water. Bring to a boil, turn down the heat and simmer gently until potatoes and fennel are cooked. Purée (with electric blender or food mill). Add the chopped apples to the puréed soup. Serve immediately.

Variation: Omit apples, if you wish.

Argyll Soup

Preparation time: 10 minutes
Cooking time: 45 minutes
Serves 4

2 large carrots
2 large onions
4 sticks celery
1 lb. potatoes
2 cloves garlic
parsley

Slice the carrots, roughly chop the onions and slice the celery. Peel and chop the potatoes and crush the garlic. Put all into a large pot and cover with water. Bring to a boil. Turn down the heat and simmer gently for 45 minutes. Purée (with electric blender or food mill). Garnish with parsley and serve immediately.

Autumn Flame Soup

Preparation time: 15 minutes
Cooking time: 25 minutes
Serves 4

1 large onion
3 large cloves garlic
1 lb. squash (or pumpkin)
4 large red bell peppers

1 lb. tomatoes, chopped
thyme
fresh green herbs (2 small bay leaves, fresh parsley or cilantro)

Chop the onion and crush the garlic. Peel and chop the squash into small chunks. Seed the peppers and chop into small pieces. Put it all into a pot and cover with water. Bring to a boil. Turn down the heat and add the chopped tomatoes, thyme and bay leaves. Simmer gently for no longer than 20 minutes. Purée (with electric blender or food mill). Serve immediately, garnished with fresh green herbs of your choice.

Beet Soup

Preparation time: 15 minutes
Cooking time: 1 hour
Serves 4

2 medium beets, unpeeled
1 large onion
1 medium carrot
2 large tomatoes
red cabbage leaves, chopped
1 bay leaf
water
1 tbsp. apple cider vinegar
juice of 1/2 lemon
herbs
yogurt
parsley

Chop beets, onion, carrot and tomatoes, without peeling (except for the onion!). Put into a large pot. Add chopped cabbage leaves and bay leaf. Cover with water and add apple cider vinegar, lemon juice and herbs. Bring to a boil, then lower heat and simmer gently for about 1 hour. When cooked, purée (with electric blender or food mill), serve with a swirl of yogurt and garnish with parsley.

Cabbage Soup

Preparation time: 10 minutes
Cooking time: 40 minutes
Serves 2-4

1 small green (or white) cabbage
2 leeks
2 potatoes, peeled
2 onions
2 sticks celery
1 clove garlic
yogurt
parsley, chopped

Coarsely chop the vegetables. Put in a pot and cover with water. Bring to a boil, lower the heat and simmer until vegetables are tender. Purée (with electric blender or food mill). Serve hot with swirls of yogurt and garnished with chopped parsley.

Broccoli Floret Soup

Preparation time: 15 minutes
Cooking time: 35 minutes
Serves 2-4

1 medium onion
6 oz. potato
1 lb. broccoli
bay leaf
yogurt

Peel and chop the onion and potato. Trim the broccoli and cut into florets. Keep a few florets to one side and put the rest into a pot with the chopped onion, potato and bay leaf, and cover with water. Bring to a boil and simmer for 20 minutes. Add the other florets and simmer for an additional 10 minutes. Remove the bay leaf. Take the whole florets from the soup and put onto a hot plate. Put the rest of the soup through the food mill. Add the other cooked florets. Reheat the soup gently. Serve immediately with a swirl of yogurt.

Carrot and Orange Soup

Preparation time: 10 minutes
Cooking time: 40 minutes
Serves 2-4

1 lb. carrots
8 oz. onions
8 oz. potatoes
juice of 1 orange
a pinch of thyme

Chop the vegetables and put them into a pot with the orange juice and the thyme, and cover with water. Bring to a boil, then simmer until vegetables are tender. Purée (with electric blender or food mill).

Cauliflower Soup

Preparation time: 10 minutes
Cooking time: 40 minutes
Serves 2-4

1 large cauliflower
1 onion
1 celery stick
10 oz. yogurt
parsley, chopped

Trim the cauliflower and break into small florets. Chop the onion and slice the celery. Put into a pot and cover with water. Bring to a boil, lower the heat and simmer gently for 30 minutes. Purée (with electric blender or food mill). Stir in the yogurt. Reheat gently before serving. Garnish with chopped parsley.

Celery, Carrot and Apple Soup

Preparation time: 10 minutes
Cooking time: 45 minutes
Serves 2-4

1 lb. celery
1 lb. carrots
8 oz. sweet apples (Pink Lady or Gala)
dill (or lemon grass)
celery leaves, chopped

Slice the celery, dice the carrots and chop the apples. Put into a large pot and cover with water. Bring to a boil, lower the heat, add the dill (or lemon grass) and simmer for 40 minutes. Purée (with electric blender or food mill). Serve immediately and garnish with chopped celery leaves.

Celery Root and Swiss Chard Soup

Preparation time: 10 minutes
Cooking time: 40 minutes
Serves 2-4

1 small celery root
1 medium leek
2 oz. Swiss chard
apple cider vinegar (or lemon juice)
parsley

Scrub and chop the celery root and leek and tear the Swiss chard into small pieces. Put into a pot with apple cider vinegar (or lemon juice) and cover with water. Bring to a boil, turn down the heat and simmer until the vegetables are soft. Purée (with electric blender or food mill). Serve hot or cold and garnish with parsley.

Corn Chowder

Preparation time: 10 minutes
Cooking time: 45 minutes
Serves 2-4

3 sticks celery
1 large potato, peeled
1 large onion
1 large green bell pepper
1 bay leaf (or a pinch of ground bay leaf)
4 ears of corn
parsley, chopped

Dice the celery, potato and onion. Remove the seeds from the pepper and dice the flesh. Put into a pot with the bay leaf and cover with water. Simmer gently until the vegetables are almost cooked. Slice the corn from the cobs and add to the soup. Cook slowly until all the vegetables are soft but not broken (about 5 minutes.). Sprinkle with the chopped parsley and serve.

Potato, Cabbage and Dill Soup

Preparation time: 10 minutes
Cooking time: 40 minutes
Serves 2-4

1 medium potato, peeled
1 medium onion
1 medium leek
white cabbage, chopped
4 tsp. dried dill
chives, chopped

Chop the potato, onion and leek. Put into a pot with the chopped cabbage and cover with water. Bring to a boil, turn down the heat and add half the dill. Simmer gently until the potatoes are cooked. Purée (with electric blender or food mill). Add the rest of the dill and reheat gently. Garnish with chopped chives and serve immediately.

Potato Soup

Preparation time: 20 minutes
Cooking time: 1-1/2 to 2 hours
Serves 4-6

1 large onion
1/2 small celery knob
2 stalks celery
2 large potatoes
1 leek
parsley
2 quarts water

Dice all vegetables. Place vegetables, parsley and water in covered saucepan and bring to boil. Lower heat and cover. Simmer 1-1/2 to 2 hours. Mash through food mill.

Sweet and Sour Cabbage Soup

Preparation time: 10 minutes
Cooking time: 15 minutes
Serves 2-4

2 medium onions
1 medium white (or green) cabbage
2 cloves garlic, crushed
2 medium tomatoes
1 tbsp. sugar
juice of 1 large lemon
3 oz. raisins
1 qt. water

Slice the onion and sweat gently in a little water for a few minutes until it starts to soften. Cut the cabbage into thin strips and add to onion, mixing well. Add crushed garlic. Chop the tomatoes and add together with the sugar, lemon juice, raisins and water. Bring to a boil and simmer until the cabbage is al dente (about 10 minutes). Serve this hearty soup as a main dish with bread followed by fruit for dessert.

Tangy Tomato Soup

Preparation time: 10 minutes
Cooking time: 25 minutes
Serves 2-4

1 lb. tomatoes
1 carrot
1 stick celery
1 onion
1 red bell pepper
little orange juice
yogurt

Chop tomatoes, carrot, celery and onion. Seed pepper and chop. Put all into a large pot and cover with water. Bring to a boil, turn down the heat and simmer until vegetables are tender. Purée (with electric blender or food mill). Add the orange juice. Reheat gently. Add a swirl of yogurt before serving.

Tomato Soup with Potato and Onion

Preparation time: 20 minutes
Cooking time: 40 minutes
Serves 3-4

2 large tomatoes
1 medium onion
2 medium potatoes
1 tsp. wine vinegar
small bay leaf

Dice all vegetables. Place all ingredients in covered saucepan, cover with water and cook over low flame for 35-40 minutes. Mash through food mill and serve hot.

Vegetables and Potatoes

Baked Pepper and Tomato Salad

Preparation time: 15 minutes
Cooking time: 30 minutes
Serves 2-4

3 red bell peppers
6 large tomatoes
1 medium red onion
3 cloves garlic
juice of 1 large lemon
3 tbsp. fresh, chopped mint
flaxseed oil

Bake the peppers and tomatoes whole at 350° F (177° C) until somewhat cooked but still firm. Skin the peppers and tomatoes, chop roughly and place in a serving dish. Finely slice the onion and very thinly slice the garlic. Add to the mixture in the dish. Add the lemon and mint. Mix well. Sprinkle with a little flaxseed oil.

Baked Potato and Parsnip Rosti*

* Rosti means "broiled" or "roasted" (i.e., top-browned)
Preparation time: 15 minutes
Cooking time: 1-1/4 hour
Serves 2

8 oz. parsnips
8 oz. potatoes
1 onion, finely chopped
2 tbsp. fresh chives, finely chopped
herbs
3-1/2 oz. yogurt
a little grated horseradish (optional)

Core the parsnips. Peel and coarsely grate the potatoes and parsnips into a large bowl. Add finely chopped onion, chives, herbs and yogurt. Mix until well combined. Put the vegetable mixture into a shallow dish and cover. Bake for 1 hour at 375° F (190° C). Remove the lid and bake a little longer until it begins to brown and the top is crispy. Serve with a crisp salad or a vegetable (or both).

Baked Potatoes

Preparation time: 5 minutes

Baked potatoes should be thoroughly washed, not scraped or peeled. Bake in a low oven at 300° F (149° C) for 2 or 2-1/2 hours or, alternatively, bake for 50 minutes to 1 hour at 350° F (177° C).

Baked Potato with Beet and Onion

Preparation time: 15 minutes
Cooking time: 1 hour

1 baking potato
1 large onion, peeled
beet, diced and cooked
yogurt
dill
1 tsp. flaxseed oil (optional)

Scrub the potato and place whole into a casserole dish with a large, peeled onion. Add a little water and bake until both are cooked. Chop the cooked onion and put into a saucepan with the diced, cooked beet. Heat through. Split open the potato and fill with the onion and beet mixture. Mix together the yogurt, dill and flaxseed oil (if using the flaxseed oil, wait until the potato is no longer steaming) and drizzle over the top. Serve with a green salad.

Baked Potato with Onion

Preparation time: 15 minutes
Cooking time: 1-1/2 hours

1 baking potato

1 onion
cooked beet
yogurt
dill

Bake the potato in its skin. Slice the onion and cook gently until beginning to soften. Dice the beet, add to the onion and warm through. When the potato is cooked, split it open and spoon in the beet mixture. Top with dollops of yogurt and sprinkle with dill. Serve with a green salad.

Baked Tomatoes

Preparation time: 10 minutes
Cooking time: 20 minutes
Serves 2

1 lb. tomatoes
1 clove garlic
1 medium onion
bread crumbs (or a handful of rolled oats)
dill
flaxseed oil

Slice the tomatoes and put into a baking dish. Crush the garlic, chop the onion and sprinkle over the tomatoes. Cover with bread crumbs (or rolled oats) and bake for about 20 minutes at 325° F (170° C). Just before serving, sprinkle with dill and flaxseed oil.

Beets

Bake at 300-350° F (149-177° C) or boil beets in their jackets.

Beets, Cooked and Creamed

Preparation time: 15 minutes
Cooking time: 60-75 minutes

3 beets, cooked and chopped

6 tbsp. yogurt
1 tbsp. fresh chives, snipped
2 tbsp. onion, finely chopped
parsley, finely chopped

Put cooked, chopped beets into a saucepan with the yogurt, chives and onion and heat gently. Put into serving dish and sprinkle with chopped parsley.

Beets with Horseradish

Preparation time: 10 minutes
Cooking time: 1 to 1-1/2 hours
Serves 2-4

6 beets
yogurt
2 tsp. horseradish
chives

Cook the beets until tender. Remove the skin and cut into quarters. Combine the yogurt and horseradish and pour over the beets. Garnish with chopped chives and serve immediately.

Bessarabian Nightmare

Preparation time: 15 minutes
Cooking time: 40 minutes
Serves 2

tomatoes
onions
red (or green) bell pepper, seeded
garlic, crushed
herbs
flaxseed oil

Skin the tomatoes. Slice the tomatoes, onions and peppers. Arrange in layers in an oven-proof dish. Sprinkle with crushed garlic and herbs.

Cook slowly, then chill and serve cold, adding a little flaxseed oil before serving. A strange name for a delicious dish!

Braised Cabbage

Preparation time: 15 minutes
Cooking time: 1 hour
Serves 2

1 lb. green cabbage
4 oz. carrots
4 oz. onion
2 sticks celery
dill seeds

Cut the cabbage into quarters. Remove the stalk, the core and any discolored leaves. Cook the cabbage in a little water in a saucepan for 10 minutes. Dice the carrots, onion and celery and put into a large oven-proof dish with very little water. Place the cabbage on top. Scatter with dill seeds. Bake covered for about 1 hour at 350° F (180° C) or until the vegetables are tender.

Braised Fennel with Orange and Tomato Sauce

Preparation time: 10 minutes
Cooking time: 30 minutes
Serves 2

1 medium head of fennel
1-1/2 lb. tomatoes
1 tbsp. tomato purée
juice of 1/2 orange
herbs
green fennel tops

Cut the fennel into quarters and remove the core. Cook gently for 8-10 minutes. Meanwhile, cook the tomatoes to a pulp and add the tomato purée, orange juice and herbs. Add the fennel and cook covered for 12-15 minutes. Garnish with fennel tops and serve.

Broccoli

Bake in a covered casserole in low oven at 300° F (149° C) with onions or a small amount of soup stock for 1-2 hours. Serve with tomato sauce.

Broccoli and Herbs

Preparation time: 20 minutes
Cooking time: 25 minutes
Serves 2

2 bunches of broccoli
4-6 cloves garlic
1/2 onion sliced
1/4 tsp. dill
1/4 cup soup stock

Peel the broccoli stems. Put garlic and onion in one pot and cook until onion becomes translucent. Add cut broccoli crowns and stems, dill and soup stock. Cook on low heat until broccoli is tender.

Broccoli, Green Beans and Pears

Preparation time: 5 minutes
Cooking time: 20 minutes
Serves 2

broccoli
green beans
2 pears

Dressing:
lemon juice (or apple cider vinegar)
flaxseed oil

Gently cook the broccoli and green beans. Allow to cool. Peel and chop the pears and put in a dish together with the broccoli and beans. Gently toss in dressing and serve with a baked potato and a mixed green salad.

Butternut Squash (Mashed)

Preparation time: 10 minutes
Cooking time: 35 minutes
Serves 2

butternut squash
1 small onion
yogurt

Peel and core chunks of butternut squash. Place in pan with one small onion. You will probably not need cooking water as the butternut squash is a "wet" vegetable. Simmer until done. Mash with enough yogurt to make smooth.

Cabbage and Tomato Hot Pot

Preparation time: 15 minutes
Cooking time: 35 minutes
Serves 2

1 small cabbage
1 onion
1 dessert apple
4 large tomatoes, skinned
yogurt
bread crumbs
parsley, chopped

Cook the cabbage gently in water until cooked but still crisp. Chop the onion, apple and skinned tomatoes and cook gently until they form a thick purée. Shred the cabbage and add to the purée. Turn into a casserole dish. Mix the yogurt with the bread crumbs and sprinkle over the top. Top-brown under the broiler to heat a little. Sprinkle with chopped parsley and serve immediately.

Carrot and Leek Bake

Preparation time: 10 minutes
Cooking time: 1-2 hours
Serves 2-4

1 lb. carrots
4 or 5 small leeks
2 medium oranges
handful of raisins

Dice or slice the carrots and slice the leeks. Put into a baking dish with the raisins. Add the juice of two oranges. Bake in a medium oven at 325° F (170° C) for 1 to 2 hours until done. If you wish, you can thicken the orange juice with corn starch to make a sauce. (Organic corn starch may be used occasionally.) Serve with a baked potato.

Carrot and Tomato Casserole

Preparation time: 15 minutes
Cooking time: 1 hour
Serves 2

8 oz. tomatoes
1/2 tbsp. chopped fresh sage (or 1/2 tsp. dried sage)
2 medium onions
1 lb. carrots

Slice or chop the tomatoes and put a layer into the bottom of a casserole dish. Add some sage. Slice the onions and place a layer on top of the tomatoes. Add another sprinkling of sage. Slice the carrot and place on top, finishing with a layer of tomato mixed with the last of the sage. Place the casserole in the oven and bake for 1 hour at 350° F (180° C) until the carrots are tender. Serve with a mixed green salad and a baked potato.

Carrots and Honey

Preparation time: 10 minutes
Cooking time: 45 minutes
Serves 1-2

carrots
soup stock
1/2 tsp. honey

Cut off the ends of the carrots and slice. Do not peel or scrape. Stew in a small amount of soup stock for 45 minutes or until tender. During the last 5 to 10 minutes of stewing, add honey for slight flavoring.

Cauliflower

Preparation time: 10 minutes
Cooking time: 45 minutes

cauliflower
2-3 tomatoes

Break cauliflower into sections. Add tomatoes, sliced and cut into chunks. Stew together for approximately 45 minutes (or until tender) on low heat.

Cauliflower and Carrot Sauce

Preparation time: 20 minutes
Cooking time: 50 minutes

1 small cauliflower
3 carrots
flaxseed oil

Separate the cauliflower florets, place them in a baking dish with a little water and cook at 250° F (121° C) for 40 minutes or until soft. When ready, drain off the water. At the same time, simmer the carrots on low heat with enough water until they are soft. Blend carrots in blender with the flaxseed oil. Pour sauce over the cooked cauliflower and place in warm oven at 250-300° F (121-149° C) (turned off) for 5-10 minutes before serving.

Chard Rolls, Stuffed

Preparation time: 40 minutes
Cooking time: 30 minutes

1/2 onion, sliced
6 medium potatoes
4 carrots
3 large cloves garlic, minced
1 bunch of chard

Cook onions and potatoes in one pot. In another pot, cook carrots and garlic. When done, purée (with electric blender or food mill) each potful separately, then mix together. Put chard leaves in very hot water, being sure not to overcook. Spread each leaf and remove tough center stem. Place purée in center of each leaf and roll tightly. Display on tray and serve with tomato sauce made with tomatoes, onion, garlic and small potato, which have been cooked and puréed.

Cooked Sweet Potato and Beet Salad

Preparation time: 10 minutes
Cooking time: 30 minutes
Serves 2

1 large (or 2 small) sweet potatoes
a few cooked small beets, sliced
arugula (or lettuce) leaves

Dressing:
yogurt
lemon juice
flaxseed oil
dill weed, dried or fresh

Cook the sweet potatoes gently in their skins until done. Allow to cool. Cut into slices and place the sweet potato and beet slices overlapping on a plate of arugula (or lettuce) leaves. Drizzle on the dressing and serve immediately.

Corn

Preparation time: 5 minutes

Corn may be baked in the husk wrapped in foil. Bake in low oven at 300° F (149° C) for 1 hour. If husked, place in boiling water for approximately 7 minutes.

Corn on the Cob Packets

Preparation time: 5 minutes
Cooking time: 1 hour
Serves 1-2

1 or 2 corn cobs
flaxseed oil
parsley, chopped

Leave the corn in its outer leaves and wrap in baking foil. Bake at 350° F (180° C) for about 1 hour. When cooked, peel back the leaves and allow to cool. Pour on some flaxseed oil to which some chopped parsley has been added. Serve as an appetizer or a side dish.

Corn with Mixed Vegetables

Preparation time: 15 minutes
Cooking time: 1 hour
Serves 2

2 ears of corn
3 stalks of celery
2 carrots
2 zucchinis squash

Husk the corn and cut the kernels off. Slice the other vegetables into small pieces. Put the corn in a baking dish and add the vegetables. Bake at 200° F (93° C) for 1 hour.

Corn with Orange Juice

Preparation time: 10 minutes

2 ears of corn
1 glass of orange juice

Husk the corn, cut off the kernels and put it in a baking dish with a lid. Bake at 250° F (121° C) until soft (approximately 25-30 minutes). Pour the corn juice off and add the orange juice. Let set 5 to 10 minutes before serving.

Creamed Corn

Preparation time: 20 minutes
Cooking time: 1-1/2 hours
Serves 2-3

3 ears of corn
1 green bell pepper, sliced

Husk corn and cut off the kernels. Put kernels from 2 ears in a blender and blend. Add the kernels from the third ear to the blended corn. Place in a baking dish and put the sliced green pepper on top and bake in the oven at 200-250° F (93-121° C) for 1-1/2 hours.

Creamed Green Beans

Preparation time: 5 minutes
Cooking time: 15 minutes
Serves 2

10 oz. whole green beans
yogurt
2 oz. onion, finely chopped

Cook the beans gently. Just before the beans are ready, gently heat the yogurt with the chopped onion. Put the beans into a warm serving dish and pour on the yogurt dressing.

Creamy Cabbage

Preparation time: 10 minutes
Cooking time: 30 minutes
Serves 2

white cabbage
1 small onion
2 tbsp. yogurt
1 tsp. dried dill tops, chopped (or crushed dill seeds)

Shred the cabbage and chop the onion. Add a little water to cook. When cooked and tender, add the yogurt mixed with the dill tops (or seeds).

Eggplant, Baked

Preparation time: 15 minutes
Cooking time: 2 hours
Serves 2

soup stock
1 onion, chopped
1 eggplant, sliced
2 tomatoes, sliced and skinned

Put some soup stock in bottom of large covered baking dish. Add onion, eggplant and tomatoes in layers. Cover and bake in a low oven at 300° F (149° C) for 2 hours.

Eggplant Fan

Preparation time: 15 minutes
Cooking time: 45 minutes
Serves 2

1 large onion

1 large eggplant
1 large firm, ripe tomato
thyme and marjoram
1 small clove garlic, chopped

Slice the onion into rings and cook gently in a thick-bottomed saucepan while preparing the other ingredients. Cut eggplant into 4 or 5 lengthwise slices, stopping 3/4 inch from either end. Slice the tomato into twice as many slices as there are cuts in the eggplant. Arrange the eggplant on top of the onions in a fan shape, and fill the cuts with the tomato slices. Sprinkle with herbs and chopped garlic. Cover and cook gently, on top of the stove, or bake gently in a low oven at 300° F (149° C) until the eggplant is soft.

Eggplant Salad

Preparation time: 15 minutes
Cooking time: 1 hour
Serves 2
1 eggplant
1 small onion
parsley
2 tomatoes
1-1/2 tbsp. vinegar
a little flaxseed oil

Bake the eggplant for about 1 hour at 350° F (180° C). Chop the onion and parsley and slice the tomatoes. Combine with the cooked eggplant. Add the vinegar and flaxseed oil.

Eggplant, Stewed

Preparation time: 20 minutes
Cooking time: 30 minutes
Serves 2

1 eggplant, cut into cubes
2 onions, chopped

3 tomatoes, peeled and chopped

Combine all ingredients in a stew pot. Stew approximately 30 minutes (until tender). Do not add water.

Fancy Garlic Potatoes

Preparation time: 5 minutes
Cooking Time: 1-1/2 to 2 hours

potatoes
flaxseed oil
garlic, crushed

Cut the potatoes into slices, not quite through to the base. Put into a casserole dish with only enough water to cover the bottom. Cook in the top of the oven at 325° F (170° C) for 1-1/2 to 2 hours or at 350° F (180° C) for 1 hour. Mix together the flaxseed oil and crushed garlic. Put the potatoes onto a serving dish and, when slightly cooled, pour on the dressing. Serve immediately.

Fennel Treat

Preparation time: 15 minutes
Cooking time: 1-2 hours
Serves 2

1 fennel bulb
1 large tomato, cut into 1/4-inch slices
2-3 cloves garlic, peeled and sliced thinly

Cut off stalks and leaves from fennel. Slice bulb in half lengthwise to give two flat halves. Rinse under running water to remove sand and put them in a baking dish with cut side up. Cover halves with tomato slices and place garlic slices on top of tomatoes. Cover the dish and bake at 250° F (121° C) for 1 to 2 hours. Serve with a baked potato and a salad of grated carrots on a bed of pretty greens.

Festive Broccoli (or Festive Green Beans)

Preparation time: 25 minutes
Cooking time: 45 minutes
Serves 2-3

1 large head broccoli (or 3-1/2 cups sliced green beans)
1 small onion, diced
1 clove garlic, minced
1 medium sweet red (or yellow) bell pepper, cut in strips
2 tsp. lemon juice (optional)
1/4 tsp. dried (or 1 tsp. fresh) dill weed

Select dark green head of broccoli with no yellowing. Cut into spears, peeling tougher stalks at base. Place onion and garlic in pot. Cover and stew on low flame for 45 minutes or until tender. Add pepper strips for the last 20 to 25 minutes of cooking. Add lemon juice just before serving (lemon will discolor broccoli if added during cooking). Sprinkle vegetables with dill and serve.

French Bean (Green Bean) Salad

Preparation time: 5 minutes
Cooking time: 10 minutes
Serves 2

French beans (green beans)
small onion, chopped
flaxseed oil
apple cider vinegar (or lemon juice)
parsley
chives

Cook the beans gently until just tender. Drain and add the chopped onion. Put into a serving dish and toss in the flaxseed oil and apple cider vinegar (or lemon juice). Add herbs and serve.

Fruited Red Cabbage

Preparation time: 10 minutes*
* Does not include soaking
Cooking time: 15 minutes
Serves 2

4 oz. raisins
4 oz. dried apricots, chopped
1 small red cabbage
2 dessert apples, cored and chopped
apple cider vinegar
a little sugar

Presoak the raisins and apricots (soak overnight in cold water, or pour boiling water over them and leave for a couple of hours until plump). Shred the red cabbage and sweat in a little water until slightly softened. Add raisins, chopped apricots and cored, chopped dessert apples. Toss in apple cider vinegar, to which a little water and sugar have been added. Pile into a bowl and serve with a baked potato.

Gerson Gardener's Pie*

*A bit like Shepherd's Pie but with vegetables instead of meat
Preparation time: 30 minutes
Cooking time: 2-1/2 hours
Serves 2-3

Topping:
1 lb. potatoes
12 oz. celery root (or sweet potato or onion)

Peel the potato and other vegetable and cut into small chunks. Add water but only about 1/2 to 2/3 the height of the vegetables. Bring to a boil and reduce to a simmer. Cook slowly until all the water is gone and the vegetables are soft, and mash. If there is a little water left in the pan, beat it into the mash mixture.

Filling:
1 small onion (or a few shallots)

2 cloves garlic, crushed
8 oz. carrots, sliced, or chipped or diced (but not diced too thickly)
8 oz. zucchini, cut into half slices, not too thin
8 oz. leeks, trimmed and sliced
2 tomatoes, skinned and chopped
1-2 tbsp. chopped parsley
herbs to taste
2 oz. bread crumbs

Prepare vegetables and put them into a saucepan in the order listed above. Cook the vegetables very gently. You may need to use a simmer plate. This could take 1 to 1-1/2 hours. Prepare topping and bread crumbs. When vegetables are cooked, stir in bread crumbs and pour the mixture into a pie plate. Top with mashed potatoes. Drag a fork over the top to decorate and bake for about 45 to 60 minutes at 350° F (180° C). Place pie plate on baking sheet in case of leakage. Serve with green vegetables and salad.

Variations: Change the contents of the pie by adding green beans, peas and/or corn when in season. Jerusalem artichokes would be also good. You could leave the leeks out of the pie and purée them (with electric blender or food mill) to add to the topping instead of the sweet potato, onion or celery root.

Gerson Roast Potatoes

Preparation time: 5 minutes
Cooking time: 1 hour

1 baking potato

Cut a baking potato in half (or, if very large, into quarters). Score across the cut surface with a knife. Put into a casserole dish with a little water to just cover the bottom. Put lid on and bake in a hot oven at 400-425° F (204-218° C) for 1 hour. Before serving, remove the lid and leave to slightly brown.

Glazed Beets

Preparation time: 25 minutes
Cooking time: 1-1/2 hours
Serves 6 to 8

9 large beets

Scrub beets and boil in 2 to 3 inches of water until tender for 1 to 1-1/2 hours. Add more water if needed. Peel in cold water. Slice or cut into bite-sized pieces.

Glaze:
2/3 cup fresh orange juice
1 tsp. cornstarch
1-1/2 tsp. apple cider vinegar
1 tsp. honey (or sugar)

Combine ingredients for glaze. Cook over low flame until thick. Add beets and mix well.

   Variation: Use 1/2 cup apple juice and 3 tsp. lemon juice in place of orange Juice.

Glazed Carrots and Turnips with Garlic

Preparation time: 10 minutes
Cooking time: 30 minutes
Serves 2

8 oz. carrots
8 oz. turnips

Dressing:
1 tbsp. lemon juice
1 clove garlic, crushed
flaxseed oil

Gently cook the carrots and turnips. Cut into thin slices and put into a serving dish. Pour on the dressing and garnish with cilantro or dill.

Glazed Carrots with Herbs and Lemon

Preparation time: 5 minutes
Cooking time: 30 minutes
Serves 2

1 lb. carrots
1 tsp. sugar
a little water
1 tbsp. lemon juice
mint
rosemary
parsley
flaxseed oil

Gently cook the carrots whole. When beginning to soften, remove from pan and cut into 2-inch sticks. Return to the saucepan with the sugar and a little water. Heat until the sugar is dissolved, the water has been absorbed and the carrots are cooked. Add the lemon juice and herbs and heat for an additional 2 minutes. Place on a warm serving dish, add flaxseed oil and serve immediately.

Glazed Carrots with Orange

Preparation time: 5 minutes
Cooking time: 30 minutes
Serves 2

1 lb. carrots
1 tbsp. sugar
juice of 1/2 orange
flaxseed oil

Gently cook the carrots whole. When beginning to soften, remove from the pan and cut into 2-inch sticks. Return to the saucepan with the sugar and orange juice. Heat until the sugar has been dissolved and the orange juice absorbed. Turn onto platter, add flaxseed oil and serve.

Green Beans in Honey and Tomato Sauce

Preparation time: 15 minutes
Cooking time: 20 minutes
Serves 2

1 lb. fine green beans

Sauce:
1 medium onion
2 cloves garlic
1 lb. tomatoes, roughly chopped
1 tsp. honey
herbs

Cut ends off the beans, cook until just tender and drain. To make the sauce, chop the onion and crush the garlic. Cook them both in a little water until just tender. When the onion is soft, add the roughly chopped tomatoes and bring to a boil. Simmer gently until sauce becomes fairly thick. Stir in the honey and herbs. Add the beans and allow to cool. Serve at room temperature.

Green Chard Rolls

Preparation time: 45 minutes
Cooking time: 2 hours

4 leaves of green chard
2 carrots
1/4 head broccoli
1/4 head cauliflower
2 small zucchini squash
1 ear of corn (cut kernels off)
1/2 cup uncooked rice

Sauce:
1-1/2 tomatoes
2 cloves garlic

Put the chard leaves in hot water long enough to wilt them so they will bend. Cut the broccoli, cauliflower, squash and corn into small pieces and put them in a pan with a little water to simmer. When cooked, drain the water off. Make a sauce in the blender with the tomatoes and garlic, and pour this sauce on top of the vegetables and uncooked rice. Place some of the vegetables/rice mixture in the center of each leaf and roll them up. Put these in a baking dish with a lid and bake in the oven at 250° F (121° C) for 1 to 1-1/2 hours.

Green Peppers

Preparation time: 10 minutes
Cooking time: 30 minutes
Serves 2-3

2-4 green peppers, sliced
2-4 onions, sliced

Stew in tightly covered pot for approximately 30 minutes. Do not add water.

Grilled Eggplant

Preparation time: 10 minutes
Cooking time: 20 minutes
Serves 1

1 eggplant
garlic
parsley, chopped
lemon (or lime) juice

Slice the eggplant lengthwise. Heat a griddle pan (preferably a "ridged" pan). When the pan is hot, turn down the heat, place the slices of egg-plant on the griddle and allow them to cook slowly. Turn over the slices and repeat. Before serving, squeeze garlic over the slices, sprinkle with chopped parsley and drizzle lemon (or lime) juice over them. This is a good main course for lunch served with new potatoes.

Variations: You can do the same thing with large slices of peppers, halves of onions or zucchini halved lengthwise.

Leek and Potato Bake

Preparation time: 15 minutes
Cooking time: 40 minutes
Serves 2

1 lb. potatoes
1 small leek
fine oats (put some regular rolled oats in the blender)

Parboil the potatoes in their skins until they are hot through and just beginning to soften. Very thinly slice the leek (using the white section only). Peel the potatoes and coarsely grate them. Mix in the leek. Put into a shallow baking dish (sprinkled at the bottom with fine oats to prevent sticking). Cook on the top shelf of the oven at 350° F (180° C) until beginning to show signs of browning. (Don't leave it for too long or it will dry out.) Serve with either cooked vegetables or a green salad and tomatoes.

Leeks (or Zucchini) à la Grecque

Preparation time: 10 minutes
Cooking time: 30 minutes
Serves 2

1 lb. leeks (or zucchini)
3 tomatoes, chopped (optional)
juice of 1 lemon
bay leaf
thyme
coriander seeds

Slice the leeks (or zucchini) into 1-inch pieces. Cook gently with chopped tomatoes (if used), lemon juice, bay leaf, thyme and coriander seeds. Serve hot or cold.

Lima Beans and Zucchini

Preparation time: 15 minutes
Cooking time: 20 minutes
Serves 1-2

1 large onion
1 clove garlic
1/2 cup soup stock
1 cup fresh lima beans
3 cups zucchini
4 medium tomatoes
1/2 tsp. cornstarch
4 sprigs fresh parsley
dash of thyme (or sage, or a pinch of dried parsley)

Mix together all ingredients except herbs. Simmer about 15 minutes (until tender). Thicken with cornstarch mixed with a little water. Just before serving, add herbs.

Lyonnaise Potatoes

Preparation time: 5 minutes
Cooking Time: 1 to 1-1/2 hours
Serves 2

1 lb. potatoes
1 large onion
2 tbsp. of water
flaxseed oil
garlic, crushed

Thickly slice the potatoes and onion. Arrange the potato slices in an oven-proof dish with a slice of onion between each potato slice. Pour on the water. Bake in oven at 300-350° F (149-177° C) until well done and beginning to brown. Allow to cool slightly, then pour on the flaxseed oil and crushed garlic. Serve immediately.

Mashed Carrot and Potato Bake

Preparation time: 10 minutes
Cooking time: 1 hour

carrots
potatoes

Cook the carrots and potatoes gently until just tender. Mash them and pile into an oven-proof dish. Decorate with diagonal fork marks and put into a hot oven at 400-425° F (204-218° C) to brown.

Mashed Potatoes

Preparation time: 20 minutes
Cooking time: 40 minutes

potatoes
1 small onion
yogurt

Peel and cube potatoes. Place in pan with one small onion and enough water to bring to a boil. Simmer until done (when there is no water left). Mash with enough yogurt to make smooth.

Mashed Potatoes and Chard

Preparation time: 15 minutes
Cooking time: 25 minutes
Serves 4

1 bunch green (or red) chard
4-5 tbsp. water (or soup stock)
3 large (or 4 medium) potatoes
6-8 oz. yogurt

Shred the chard and put in pan. Add water (or soup stock) and start to boil. When boiling, turn down to simmer. Meanwhile, peel potatoes, cube and place on top of the chard. Let simmer until potatoes are soft and done. Remove any remaining water and add yogurt. Mash all together. Add a little more yogurt if the mixture is too dry.

Variation: The same recipe can be used with kale. When using kale, strip out central stems before shredding into pan.

Mashed Potatoes Gerson Style

Preparation time: 10 minutes
Cooking time: 35 minutes

potatoes, peeled and cut into pieces
onion, peeled and chopped small

Place potatoes and onions in a pot. Add just enough water to reach the vegetables half-way up. Cover, bring to boil and simmer until potatoes are cooked. (Most of the cooking water will probably be gone.) Mash potatoes and onions using some (or all) of the cooking water. If not enough moisture, add some soup stock.

Variations: Add any herb of your choice, finely chopped. Parsley is very good; mint and dill will also work.

Oven-Browned Potatoes

Preparation time: 5-10 minutes

potatoes

Cut the potatoes like French fries (or in small cubes, or in thin slices) and brown on an oven tray in the oven. They will brown at a surprisingly low heat (300° F or 149° C), if left in long enough. Depending on the variety of potato, they can brown very quickly and puff up at high heat (425° F or 218° C). They can also be browned under the broiler, but watch them to avoid burning. This is meant to be an occasional treat!

Parsley Potatoes

potatoes
parsley, chopped
flaxseed oil

Boil several potatoes in their skins until done. Remove the peel and roll in some chopped parsley after slightly brushing with flaxseed oil.

Parsnips and Sweet Potatoes

Preparation time: 10 minutes
Cooking time: 40 minutes
Serves 2-4

1 lb. parsnips
1 lb. sweet potatoes
sprig of fresh rosemary

Cut the parsnips and sweet potatoes into wedges, leaving the skins intact. Put into a baking dish with a little water to cover the bottom. Add a sprig of rosemary. Cover and bake in a medium oven at 325° F (170° C) until just cooked. Serve with a baked potato.

Patate alla Francesca

Preparation time: 5 minutes
Cooking time: 40 minutes

new potatoes
tomatoes
fresh rosemary sprigs
garlic

Bake new potatoes in a covered dish at 300-350° F (149-177° C) with chopped or sliced tomatoes, fresh rosemary sprigs and plenty of garlic. Serve with lemon wedges and a green salad.

Piemontese Peppers

Preparation time: 10 minutes
Cooking time: 1 hour
Serves 2

2 tomatoes
2 red bell peppers

2 cloves garlic, sliced
herbs

Skin the tomatoes. Halve the peppers and remove the seeds (but not the stalks). Place the peppers skin-side down in a baking dish. Place slices of garlic inside each pepper half and top each with half a skinned tomato. Bake covered at 350° F (180° C) until tender and sweet (about 1 hour). Serve hot or cold, sprinkled with herbs.

Potato and Celery Root Lyonnaise

Preparation time: 15 minutes
Cooking Time: 1-1/2 to 2 hours
Serves 2

1 small to medium onion
1 small to medium celery root, scrubbed (and, if necessary, peeled)
1 medium potato, scrubbed

Slice all the ingredients thinly. Arrange in layers (onion, celery root and, potato) in a small soufflé dish. Add a very little amount of water. Bake for 1-1/2 to 2 hours at 325° F (170° C). The top layer will get crisp while the lower layers should be soft. Serve with green vegetable of your choice and a salad.

Potato Cakes

Preparation time: 25 minutes
Cooking time: 30 minutes
Serves 2-4

1 lb. potatoes
1 large carrot
1 green bell pepper
1 stick of celery
fine oats (put some regular rolled oats in the blender)

Parboil the potatoes in their skins until they are hot through and just beginning to soften. Put through the food mill. (This will also get rid of the skin.) Cut carrot into thin matchsticks. Chop the green pepper and celery. Add these to the potato purée and form into small cakes. Coat with oats and bake in the oven at 325° F (170° C) on a baking sheet sprinkled with fine oats to prevent sticking.

Potatoes and Carrots, Westphalian Style

Preparation time: 10 minutes
Cooking time: 35 minutes
Serves 4

6-8 small (or 4-5 large carrots) carrots
3 medium (or 2 large) potatoes
1 large onion
3-4 tbsp. of soup stock

Slice carrots into pan. Peel and slice potatoes and chop onion. Add all together in pan with soup stock. Let simmer until done, adding a bit more soup stock, if necessary. When done, no liquid should remain in pan.

Potatoes Anna

Preparation time: 20 minutes
Cooking time: 1 to 1-1/2 hours
Serves 2

onion, cooked
1 lb. potatoes
garlic, crushed
yogurt
parsley, finely chopped

Sweat the onions in a covered saucepan over very low heat for approximately 1 hour. Using a 10-inch flan (or quiche) tin with at least 1-inch sides, place a layer of sweated onions on the bottom of the tin. Sprinkle with a little water to stop the onions from sticking. Very thinly slice the potatoes and layer them in the dish on top of the onions. Sprinkle with crushed garlic and some of the yogurt. Add an additional two layers, again sprinkling with garlic and yogurt. Press down each layer and make sure the potatoes overlap each other very slightly so there are no spaces. Cover the dish (e.g., by using a base from a larger, loose-bottomed cake tin). Bake at 350° F (180° C) for about 1 to 1 to 1-1/2 hours or until the potatoes feel soft when pierced with a knife. Check the potatoes while cooking; if they look too dry, add a little more yogurt. To serve, turn the potato cake out of its dish and sprinkle with finely chopped parsley.

Potato Puffs

Preparation time: 5 minutes
Cooking time: 45-50 minutes

baking potato

Take a baking potato and cut it into 1/2-inch slices. Place the slices on the oven rack and, without any addition, bake at high heat (425° F (218° C)) to puff. Turn over and lower heat to 325° F (163° C) with oven door cracked open. Bake for another 20 minutes. The slices puff up and become crisp and tasty, almost like fried potatoes. Done when shiny brown on both sides. This is marginal food, so eat it occasionally.

Potato Salad

Preparation time: 10 minutes
Cooking time: 20 minutes
Serves 2

1 lb. small new potatoes
large sprig of mint
1 tbsp. fresh parsley

Dressing:
4 oz. yogurt
a little flaxseed oil
2 cloves garlic, crushed

Scrub the potatoes and put in a saucepan with a little water. Gently simmer until cooked but still firm. While the potatoes are still hot, slice them and put into a warm dish. Pour over the dressing. Finish by sprinkling fresh chopped mint and parsley.

Quick Bake Potatoes

Preparation time: 5 minutes
Cooking time: 1 hour

potatoes
flaxseed oil

Cut potatoes in half lengthwise and score cut surfaces with diagonal lines crossing each other (like lattice work). They will cook in about half the time (about 50 minutes) in the oven at 300-350° F (149-177° C); when cool enough, the surfaces can be coated with flaxseed oil.

Quick Tomatoes and Zucchini

Preparation time: 5 minutes
Cooking time: 30 minutes
Serves 2

2 medium tomatoes
1 clove garlic, crushed
1/4 to 1/2 tsp. sugar (optional)
1 medium zucchini

Slice the tomatoes and place in the bottom of a saucepan, along with the crushed garlic and sugar (if using). Slice the zucchini and place on top. Set on a gentle heat. When the tomatoes begin to cook, stir, cover and cook for about 20 minutes.

Ratatouille

Preparation time: 15 minutes
Cooking time: 1 hour
Serves 2-4

8 oz. onions
8 oz. green/red/yellow bell peppers

8 oz. eggplant
4 tomatoes
1 clove garlic
2 tsp. apple cider vinegar
marjoram

Slice the onions and place in a baking dish. Seed and thinly slice the peppers. Add to the dish. Cut the eggplants in quarters lengthwise and then into 1/4-inch slices and add. Chop the tomatoes and finely chop the garlic clove. Add to the dish together with the apple cider vinegar and a sprinkling of marjoram. Cook very gently in the oven at 325° F (170° C) until well done. Can also be cooked on top of the stove.

Red Cabbage

Preparation time: 25 minutes
Cooking time: 1 hour
Serves 2-3

1/2 red cabbage, shredded
3 tsp. vinegar
3 large onions, chopped
2 bay leaves
a little soup stock
3 apples, peeled and grated
1 tsp. sugar

Combine cabbage, vinegar, onions, bay leaves and soup stock in a pan. Stew over low heat for approximately 1 hour. At the 1/2-hour mark, add apples and sugar.

Red Cabbage and Apple Casserole

Preparation time: 15 minutes
Cooking time: 1-1/2 hours
Serves 2

medium red cabbage
apples (cooking or green)

juice of 1 orange
apple cider vinegar
maple syrup

Shred the red cabbage and slice the apple. Place layers of red cabbage and apple in a casserole dish. Pour over the orange juice, apple cider vinegar and maple syrup. Cover with a tight-fitting lid and bake at 350° F (180° C) for about 1-1/2 hours or until tender. Stir and serve. Almost better as a reheated leftover!

Red Kuri Squash with Vegetables

Preparation time: 15 minutes
Cooking time: 30 minutes
Serves 2-4

1 red kuri squash
1 tbsp. water
1 small sweet potato, cooked
1 small zucchini, cooked
1 red (or green) bell pepper, cooked
1 tomato, peeled
onion (or garlic) powder
fresh herbs

Cut the red kuri squash in half. This is easily done with a very sharp, pointed knife. Scoop out the seeds, leaving the rest of the red flesh intact. Stand upright in an oven-proof dish to which the water has been added. Cover and bake at 300-350° F (149-177° C) until cooked (about 30 minutes; test by inserting a knife into the flesh). If there is enough room, the other vegetables could be cooked in the same dish. Otherwise, bake them in a separate dish in the same way, or cook them gently on top of the stove in a saucepan. When cooked, pile the vegetables into the squash halves. Sprinkle with onion (or garlic) powder or fresh herbs. Serve with a colorful mixed salad.

Roasted Zucchini and Pepper Salad

Preparation time: 10 minutes
Cooking time: 30 minutes
Serves 2

1 lb. small zucchini
2 red bell peppers
yogurt
3 tbsp. mint, roughly chopped

Dressing:
2 tbsp. lemon juice
2 cloves garlic, crushed
flaxseed oil

Cut the ends off the zucchini and cut in half lengthwise. Seed the peppers and cut into quarters. Put the zucchini and peppers skin-side up on a baking tray. Bake in oven at 325° F (170° C) for about 1/2 hour. When cooked and tender, cool slightly and cut into 1-inch lengths. Put into a serving dish, pour on the dressing and add the chopped mint. Serve with a smattering of cottage cheese (unsalted and uncreamed or fat-free).

Rolled Chard Parcels

Preparation time: 10 minutes
Cooking time: 30 minutes

chard leaves
green onions
snow peas
asparagus
broccoli
julienne of carrots
red chard stems

Set aside the chard leaves. Gently cook the green onions, snow peas, asparagus, broccoli, carrots and red chard stems in very little water and then chop them. Blanch the chard leaves. Fill with the cooked vegetable medley and form into "packets." Cook briefly in the oven at 300-350° F (149-177° C) for a few minutes until heated through. Serve hot or cold.

Root Vegetable Rosti*

* Rosti means "broiled" or "roasted" (i.e., top-browned)
Preparation time: 10 minutes
Cooking time: 1 hour
Serves 2

1 small onion
8 oz. potatoes
4 oz. carrots
4 oz. swede (rutabaga)
dill

Thinly slice the onion and cook by "sweating" in a little water. Meanwhile, gently cook the potatoes, carrots and swede (rutabaga). Drain thoroughly and, when cool enough to handle, coarsely grate into a bowl. Stir in the softened onion and dill. Put the mixture into an oven-proof dish. Bake for about 1/2 hour in the top of the oven at 350° F (180° C) or until cooked and slightly browning. Serve immediately.

Sauté of Sweet Potatoes

Preparation time: 15 minutes
Cooking time: 20 minutes
Serves 2-4

4 medium sweet potatoes
juice of 1 orange
a little sugar
flaxseed oil

Cook the sweet potatoes in their skins until just cooked. Allow to cool slightly, then cut into cubes. Put orange juice and sugar into a saucepan with the sweet potatoes. Heat gently but don't let the mixture boil. Put into a serving dish and allow to cool a little. Add the flaxseed oil, toss and serve immediately with fresh parsley (or chives) and a green salad.

Scalloped Potatoes (Without Yogurt)

Preparation time: 15 minutes
Cooking time: 1-2 hours

1 onion
potatoes
tomato, sliced
marjoram and/or thyme

Place a whole chopped onion in the bottom of a glass baking dish. Slice potatoes and place one layer on top of the onion. Add a layer of sliced tomato on top, then another layer of sliced or chopped onion. Sprinkle with a dash of marjoram and/or thyme and bake in a low oven at 300° F (149° C) for 1 to 2 hours or until done.

Scalloped Potatoes (With Yogurt)

Preparation time: 15 minutes
Cooking time: 1 to 1-1/2 hours
Serves 2

1 lb. potatoes
1 small onion
1 clove garlic
yogurt

Cook the potatoes gently until just cooked but firm. Slice thinly. Finely chop the onion and garlic. Arrange the slices of potato, layered with onion and garlic, in a pie dish. Pour over the yogurt and bake at 350° F (180° C) for 1 to 1-1/2 hours or until well cooked and beginning to brown on top.

Spinach

Preparation time: 10 minutes
Cooking time: 20 minutes

spinach
onions, chopped

After cutting off roots, wash spinach 3 to 4 times. Put in large, tightly covered pot that has a layer of chopped onions on the bottom of the pan. Do not add water. Stew over a low flame until spinach wilts. Pour off excess juice. Serve chopped with slice of lemon.

Spinach (or Chard) with Tomato Sauce

Preparation time: 15 minutes
Cooking time: 15 minutes

spinach (or chard)
lemon grass
sprig of rosemary
allspice (optional)

Cook the spinach (or chard) with some lemon grass and a sprig of rosemary. Add a pinch of allspice, if desired. Thinly cut the ribs of the spinach (or chard) and cook the leaves. Serve with tomato sauce.

Stuffed Eggplant

Preparation time: 20 minutes
Cooking time: 1 hour
Serves 2

1 eggplant
4 oz. tomatoes
1 medium onion
1 clove garlic, crushed
1 tbsp. fresh chopped parsley

Place the whole eggplant in a large saucepan and cover with boiling water. Let stand for 10 minutes, then plunge into cold water. Meanwhile, in another saucepan, very gently cook the tomatoes for 5 minutes. Press through sieve to get rid of the skins and set aside the pulp. Cut the cooled eggplants in half lengthwise. Scoop out the pulp, leaving a 1/2-inch thick outer shell. Chop the eggplant pulp and set aside. Place the eggplant shells in a shallow baking dish with just a little water in the bottom to prevent sticking. Bake for 30 minutes at 350° F (180° C). Sauté onion and crushed garlic in a small amount of boiling water until tender. Stir in the parsley. Add the sieved tomato pulp and chopped eggplant pulp, and cook for 20 minutes on moderate heat until it thickens. Spoon this mixture into the cooked eggplant shells. Keep warm in the oven until serving, or leave to cool and serve cold.

Stuffed Mixed Vegetables

Preparation time: 25 minutes
Cooking time: 30 minutes
Serves 2-4

1 zucchini
1 eggplant
2 small onions, chopped
garlic, crushed
marjoram
1 green (or red) bell pepper
soup stock

Cut the zucchini and eggplant in half, scoop out the pulp of the eggplant (carefully leaving a shell) and cook with the onion, crushed garlic and marjoram. Cut the peppers in half and take out the seeds. Stuff the eggplant, zucchini and peppers with the mixture and put in a shallow baking dish on a layer of onion rings. Bake at 300-350° F (149-177° C) until the pepper is done. Add a little soup stock if the dish seems to be getting dry. Serve with tomato sauce.

Stuffed Pepper

Preparation time: 10 minutes
Cooking time: 50 minutes
Serves 1

red (or green) bell pepper
leftover mixed, chopped vegetables
tomatoes, sliced

Halve the pepper and seed it. Place it open-side up in an oven-proof dish. Stuff leftover mixed, chopped vegetables into pepper halves. Place slices of tomato over the top. Cook at 350° F (180° C) for 40 to 50 minutes or until the pepper is soft. Serve with broccoli or another very green vegetable.

Variation: For a change from baked potato, serve with "Potato Puffs" (p. 277).

Stuffed Squash

Preparation time: 30 minutes*
* Does not include presoaking
Serves 4-6

3-4 acorn squash
1/2 cup onion, diced
1/2 cup celery, diced
1/2 cup carrot, diced
1-1/4 cup cooked brown rice
1/2 cup lentils sprouted
1/4 cup raisins (or chopped prunes), presoaked and drained
3 tsp. fresh parsley, minced
1/2 tsp. rubbed sage
1/2 tsp. thyme
1 large clove garlic, crushed

Slice squash lengthwise and remove seeds. Presoak raisins (or chopped prunes) (soak overnight in cold water, or pour boiling water over them and leave for a couple of hours until plump) and add. Combine remaining ingredients and fill squash halves. Cover and bake at 300-325° F (149-163° C) for 1-1/2 hours or until squash is tender. Delicious with carrot sauce in "Cauliflower and Carrot Sauce" (p. 256).

Variation: For a delicious mild flavor, try using 6-8 whole garlic cloves. Crushing the fresh garlic releases its strong aromatic oils, whereas using it uncut imparts a mild taste.

Sweet Potato and Apple Bake

Preparation time: 15 minutes
Cooking time: 1 hour
Serves 2

8 oz. sweet potatoes
2 eating apples, sliced
a little water
a little sugar
allspice (optional)

Cook the sweet potatoes gently in their skins until just cooked. Allow to cool. Slice and put into a baking dish alternating with layers of apple. Over each layer, sprinkle some water and a little sugar (and allspice, if using). Bake at 300-350° F (149-177° C) covered for 20 minutes, then remove cover and bake for an additional 10 minutes. Serve as a main dish with a salad (if omitting the allspice) or as a dessert (if using allspice).

Tangy Sweet and Sour Casserole

Preparation time: 20 minutes
Cooking Time: 1-1/2 to 2 hours
Serves 2

1 large (or 2 small) cooking apples
a few slices of leek
1 small onion
1 small sweet potato
1 small parsnip
bay leaf
1 tomato
1 large clove garlic
thyme
1 small zucchini, sliced

Peel and slice the apple, and arrange half the slices in the bottom of a casserole dish. Slice the leek and arrange on top of the apple. Peel and slice the onion and add a layer. Slice the sweet potato, core and chop the parsnip and add a further layer, intermingling with the rest of the apple slices. Put a bay leaf in the middle of the casserole. Skin the tomato and slice, adding a further layer to the casserole. Crush the garlic and sprinkle over the tomato with the thyme and add a layer of sliced zucchini. Cover and bake in the oven at 350° F (180° C) for 1-1/2 to 2 hours.

Vegetable Casserole

Preparation time: 20 minutes
Cooking time: 1 hour

onions
tomatoes
leeks
potatoes
zucchinis
peppers
carrots

Using a heavy saucepan with a tight-fitting lid, slice a layer of either onions, tomatoes or leeks (or all three) and put layer in the bottom of the pan. Take an assortment of sliced, chopped or cubed vegetables and put in layers until about 3/4 full. Add a little water if needed. Cook gently for 45 minutes or until done.

Winter Vegetable Casserole

Preparation time: 20 minutes
Cooking time: 2 hours
Serves 2

sweet potato
parsnip
swede (rutabaga)
celery root
celery stalks
fennel root

tomatoes
Brussels sprouts
bay leaves
water (or soup stock)
fresh parsley, chopped

Chop, slice or dice any or all of the above ingredients (with the exception of the Brussels sprouts and parsley). Put into a large casserole dish with the bay leaves and very little water (or soup stock) to stop the vegetables from sticking. Cover and cook slowly at 325° F (170° C) for 1-1/2 hours. Trim and halve the Brussels sprouts, add to the casserole and continue to cook for another 1/2 hour. Sprinkle with fresh, chopped parsley just before serving.

Zucchini and Potato Bake

Preparation time: 20 minutes
Cooking time: 1-1/2 hours
Serves 2

1 lb. zucchini
1 lb. potatoes
2 medium onions
2 cloves garlic
10 oz. yogurt
fresh parsley, chopped

Finely slice the zucchini, potatoes and onions. Place alternate layers of zucchini, potatoes and onions in a casserole dish, adding a sprinkling of crushed garlic between the layers. Cook in the oven at 300-350° F (149-177° C) for about 1-1/2 hours. Meanwhile, crush the second garlic clove and add to the yogurt. When the dish is cooked, remove from the oven and spread the yogurt mixture on top. Sprinkle chopped fresh parsley over the top and serve immediately.

Zucchini with Garlic and Parsley

Preparation time: 15 minutes
Cooking time: 35 minutes
Serves 2

1 lb. zucchini
3 tbsp. parsley
2 cloves garlic
juice of 1 lemon
flaxseed oil

Chop both ends off the zucchinis and cook whole. While they are cooking, finely chop the parsley and crush the garlic. Mix with the lemon juice and flaxseed oil. Put into a serving bowl. When the zucchinis are cooked, halve lengthwise (if small) or slice thickly (if large). While still hot, add to the serving bowl and toss in the mixture. Serve immediately with oven-roasted bell peppers, a baked potato and a green salad.

Zucchini with Mint

Preparation time: 10 minutes
Cooking time: 30 minutes
Serves 2

4 small zucchinis
2 tbsp. apple cider vinegar
2 tbsp. water
2 tbsp. chopped mint

Cook the zucchinis gently until just cooked but firm. Cut both ends off, then cut diagonally into thin slices. Put into a small casserole dish. Mix the apple cider vinegar, water and chopped mint and pour over the sliced zucchini. Bake gently in the oven at 300° F (149° C) until warmed through. Cool and serve with a baked potato and a green salad.

Desserts

Applesauce, Cooked

Preparation time: 10 minutes
Cooking time: 15-20 minutes
Serves 2

3 medium apples, pared, cored and sliced
honey (or sugar), if needed

Put apple slices in saucepan half covered with cold water. Add honey (or sugar) to taste. Boil about 15 minutes or until soft. Put through food mill.

Applesauce, Fresh

Preparation time: 10 minutes

3 medium apples, pared, cored and sliced
honey (or sugar)

Add honey (or sugar) to taste. Run apples through the grinder portion of the juicer.

Apple Spice Cake

1/4 cup honey (or maple syrup)
1 cup fresh applesauce
1-1/2 cups oat flour
3/4 cup triticale flour
3/4 cup sugar
a pinch of allspice
a pinch of mace
1/4 tsp. coriander
2 cups raisins (or chopped dates)

Crumb topping:
2/3 cup rolled oats
1/3 cup maple syrup (or honey)

a pinch of allspice
a pinch of mace

Combine honey (or maple syrup), applesauce and flours. Sift together sugar, allspice, mace and coriander. Add raisins (or dates). Combine wet and dry ingredients. Pour into oblong bake pan. For crumb topping, buzz oats briefly in blender to make a finer flake. Mix spices with oats. Mix in enough maple syrup (or honey) to make a crumbly mixture. When the crumb topping is made, sprinkle on top. Bake at 325° F (163° C) for 40 minutes or until cake tests done. Serve with a spoonful of fresh applesauce or yogurt.

Apple-Sweet Potato Pudding

Preparation time: 20 minutes
Cooking time: 30 minutes
Serves 2-3

1 sweet potato, boiled, peeled and sliced
1 apple, raw, peeled and sliced
1 tsp. raisins
1/2 cup bread crumbs
1 tsp. sugar
1/2 cup orange juice
3 tsp. yogurt

Place sweet potato slices in baking dish with apple slices and raisins spread with bread crumbs, sugar and orange juice. Bake in oven at 350° F (177° C) for 30 minutes. Serve hot with yogurt.

Banana (Broiled)

Preparation time: 5 minutes
Cooking time: 10 minutes
Serves 1

1 banana
1 tsp. sugar
lemon juice

Cut banana in half lengthwise and add sugar and a few drops of lemon. Place in pan and broil under low flame in its skin for 10 minutes. Serve hot.

Cherries (Stewed)

Preparation time: 10 minutes
Cooking time: 12 minutes
Serves 2

1/2 lb. cherries, stemmed
1 tsp. potato starch
2 tsp. cold water
2 tsp. sugar (if needed)

Place cherries in saucepan with water to cover. Cook 10 minutes over low flame. Add potato starch dissolved in cold water. Add to boiling cherries. Cook 2 minutes longer. Chill and serve. (Cherries are particularly healthful and are best enjoyed raw.)

Currants

Preparation time: 5 minutes
Serves 1-2

1/4 lb. red currants
3 tsp. sugar
yogurt

Clean currants thoroughly before removing stems. Place in dish, add sugar and serve. Yogurt, sweetened with sugar, may be used for sauce.

Fruit Combination

Preparation time: 5 minutes
Cooking time: 13-15 minutes
Serves 3

3 cups fresh cherries and apricots, halved, sliced and pitted
2 cups water

1/2 cup sugar

2 tsp. cornstarch, dissolved in 1/3 cup cold water

Place fruit with water and sugar in saucepan. Boil gently and slowly for 10 minutes. Add cornstarch. Cook 3 minutes longer. Cool and serve.

Glazed Pear Halves

Preparation time: 15 minutes
Cooking time: 15 minutes
Serves 4

4-5 ripe pears

4 oz. water

4 tbsp. honey (or sucanat, an organic dried cane sugar)

Cut ripe pears into halves and core. Add water to honey (or sucanat) and mix well. Place pear halves in baking dish and pour sugar mixture over them. Bake in slow oven at 250° F (121° C) until done. Baste with juice if necessary.

Oatmeal Cake

Preparation time: 20 minutes
Cooking time: 45 minutes
Serves 6

4 cups oatmeal (dry oats)

2 carrots, grated or blended

honey and raisins (as desired)

Combine all the above ingredients in a baking dish. Put in the oven without a lid and bake for 45 minutes at 250° F (121° C). Serve with yogurt.

Peaches

Preparation time: 15 minutes
Cooking time: 10 minutes
Serves 1-2

1/2 lb. peaches, skinned
2 tsp. sugar

Place peaches in boiling water for 1/2 minute, drain and peel. Cut in halves. Remove pits and place in saucepan with boiling water to half cover fruit level. Cover. Simmer for 10 minutes. Cool. Add sugar and serve chilled.

Pears

Preparation time: 5 minutes
Cooking time: 20 minutes
Serves 1

1 large pear, peeled, cored and halved
1 tsp. sugar

Place pear halves in saucepan with water to half cover. Add sugar and cook for 20 minutes

Plums

Preparation time: 10 minutes
Cooking time: 15 minutes
Serves 1

1/2 lb. plums
2 tsp. sugar

Cut plums in half and remove pits (or plums can be cooked whole). Place in saucepan with water to cover. Cook 15 minutes. Remove, cool and add sugar. Serve chilled.

Prune and Banana Whip

Preparation time: 10 minutes*
*Does not include presoaking
Cooking time: 10 minutes
Serves 2

1 cup dried prunes
2 small bananas, mashed
juice of 1/4 lemon
1 tsp. sugar

Presoak the prunes (soak overnight in cold water, or pour boiling water over them and leave for a couple of hours until plump) and cook for 10 minutes. Whip all ingredients together thoroughly and put in refrigerator for 1 hour. May be served in slices decorated with sweetened yogurt.

Prunes and Apricots (Dried)

Preparation time: 5 minutes*
* Does not include presoaking
Cooking time: 15 minutes
Serves 2

1/2 lb. prunes
1/2 lb. apricots
1/3 cup barley

Presoak the prunes and apricots (soak overnight in cold water, or pour boiling water over them and leave for a couple of hours until plump). Use same water and let boil for 10 minutes or until barley is done. Cool and serve.

Gerson Materials Resource List

A number of items used routinely in the course of the Gerson treatment are not readily available in drug stores, pharmacies, food stores, etc. In order to help persons using this treatment, we suggest the following list. Sources frequently need to be updated. An updated list will be found on the Internet (www.Gerson.org).

Recommended Juicers

See "Juice Machines," p. 124, in Chapter 14, "The Gerson Household."

Also please note that citrus juices (orange or grapefruit) must be extracted with a reamer type, electric or hand operated machine, in order to avoid pressing the skins of oranges, lemons, or grapefruit.

The best, and most expensive, juicer for the Gerson Therapy is the Norwalk Hydraulic Press Juicer. All juicers can be configured for export with 220-240 volts.

Contact: Richard Boger, Norwalk Factory Representative
U.S. phone: (800) 405-8423
Overseas phone: +1 (760) 436-9684
Fax: (760) 436-9651
Website: www.nwjcal.com

Information on the Gerson Therapy, Books, Booklets, DVDs , CDs and more

Gerson Health Media
316 Mid Valley Center, #230
Carmel, CA 93923
Phone: (530) 529-1100
Email: info@gersonmedia.com
Website: www.gersonmedia.com

The Gerson Institute
Mailing address:
P.O. Box 161358
San Diego, CA 92176

Address:
4631 Viewridge Avenue
San Diego, CA 92123

Local phone: (858) 694-0707
Toll free inside the United States:
(888) 4-GERSON / (888) 443-7766
Fax: (858) 694-0757
E-mail: info@gerson.org
Website: www.gerson.org

Healing the Gerson Way is now available in Arabic, Croatian, German, Hungarian, Italian, Japanese, Korean, Polish, Romanian, Slovenian, Spanish, Chinese and French, with other languages to follow.

Dr. Max Gerson: Healing the Hopeless is now available in German. Please check for availability with the Gerson Institute.

Margaret Straus (Italy)
E-mail: Associazione.Gerson@gmail.com

Gerson Health Centre, Hungary
2098 Dobogókö
Téry Ödön u. 18
Hungary
Phone: +36 30 64 26 341
E-mail: info@gerson.hu
Website: www.gerson.hu

Hungarian Gerson Support Group
Egészségforrás Alapítvány
1092 Budapest IX
Raday u. 37 III.1, Hungary
Phone: +36 1 217 1360
E-mail: info@efa.t-online.hu

Gerson Treatment Medical Supplies

Online

Statmx.com
416 W. San Ysidro Blvd., Suite L-229
San Diego, CA 92173-2450
Phone: (619) 428-4574
Fax: (619) 428-4474
E-mail: info@statmx.com

S.T.A.T., S.A.
Apartado Postal No. 404,
Admon. de Correos
Playas de Tijuana, B.C.N. 22501
Mexico
Phone: +(52) 664 680-1103 (Mexico)
Fax: +(52) 664 680-2529 (Mexico)

or

SERVICIOS
Apartado Postal No. 404
Admon. de Correos
Playas de Tijuana, B.C.N. 22501 Mexico
Phone: +(52) 664 680-1103 (Mexico)
Fax: +(52) 664 680-2529 (Mexico)

Checks, Bank drafts, International Bank draft, MasterCard, Visa and Discover cards accepted.

Statmx.com supplies Gerson medications; use SERVICIOS as supplier of prescription items, such as needles, crude liver (when available), and B_{12}.

ISHI: Director: Ana Ma. Orozco
524 W. Calle Primera, Suite 1005-E
San Ysidro, CA 92173
To order all Gerson supplies: 866-LAB-ISHI or (866) 522-4744
Phone: (619) 428-6085
Fax: (619) 428-6095
E-mail: anama@sbcglobal.net

The Key Company
1313 West Essex Avenue
St. Louis, MO 63122
Phone: (800) 325-9592
Fax: (800) 455-0306
E-mail: info@thekeycompanyusa.com
Website: www.thekeycompanyusa.com

For those that want to implement Gerson Therapy or follow a Gerson lifestyle, who are not located near a grocery store or farm co-op that offers organic produce or supplies, there is an option that may be right for you: The Green Polka Dot Box™. Please visit www.greenpolkadotbox.com/gersonmedia.

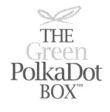
THE Green PolkaDot BOX™

The Green Polka Dot Box is poised to become the largest and most influential organic buying community ever created. By combining the delivery of healthy and natural organic foods to health-minded consumers at affordable prices, with the ability to ship to every zip code, The Green Polka Dot Box has put an end to the "organic deserts" that exist throughout America.

Enema Supplies

Gerson Health Media
14370 Del Oro Court
Red Bluff, CA 96080
Phone: (530) 529-1100
Email: info@gersonmedia.com
Website: www.gersonmedia.com

Optimal Health Network
3714 Atwood Ave.
Madison, WI 53714
Office hours: M-F 10 a.m. to 5 p.m. (Central Time)
Phone: (608) 242-0200
E-mail: Kristina@optimalhealthnetwork.com
Website: www.optimalhealthnetwork.com

Royal Blue Organics/Café MAM
P.O. Box 21123
Eugene, OR 97402
Phone: (888) Café-Mam or (888) 223-3626
(541) 338-9585
Website: www.cafemam.com

Bread

Dimpflmeier Bakery
26-36 Advance Rd.
Toronto ON M8Z 2T4 Canada

Phone: (416) 236-2701
E-mail for sales: orders@dimpflmeierbakery.com

For more information, Google them at "Dimpflmeier." They clearly state that the bread is organic, 100% rye and salt free. They make several other types of bread, so be sure to specify what it is that you want.

Source of Pure, All-Natural Supplements for Gerson Patients

Time Honored Formulas
37 Main Street, Box 1196 / 139 Second Hill Road
New Milford, CT 06776
Phone: (855) 216-3002
Fax: (860) 355-8976
E-mail: nutricons6@sbcglobal.net

Information about Fresh Organic Produce

Center for Science in the Public Interest
(provides a list of U.S. mail order businesses that sell organic food)
1220 L Street NW, Suite 300
Washington, DC 20005
Phone: (202) 332-9110
Fax: (202)265-4954
Website: www.cspinet.org

Co-Op America
(publishes National Green Page listing businesses offering organic food)
1612 K Street NW, Suite 600
Washington, DC 20006
Phone: (800) 584-7336
Website: www.greenamerica.org

Flaxseed Oil

Omega Nutrition
(state that you are a Gerson patient to receive a discount)
6515 Aldrich Rd.
Bellingham, WA 98226
Orders: (800) 661-FLAX / (800) 661-3529
Fax: (604) 253-4228
Email: info@omeganutrition.com
Website: www.omeganutrition.com

Water Distillers

The Cutting Edge
Jules Klapper, Owner
P.O. Box 4158
Santa Fe, NM 87502
Phone: (800) 497-9516 or (505) 982-2688
Website: http://cutcat.com

H2Only Distillers
J.C. Smith, Owner
216 Patterson Avenue
Butler, PA 16001
Phone: (724) 287-5555 or (800) 4-H2ONLY
Website: www.h2only.us

Renewed Health Supply
2101 Regents Park Lane
Greensboro, NC 27455
Phone: (800) 678-9151 (from United States only) or (336) 510-9915
E-mail: ryan@renewedhealth.com
Website: www.renewedhealth.com

Pure Water, Inc.
Aqua Clean MD-4
3725 Touzalin Avenue / P.O. Box 83226
Lincoln, NE 68507
(contact main office for local Aqua Clean distributor)
Phone: (402) 467-9300
Fax: (402) 467-9393

Shower Filters

The Cutting Edge
Jules Klapper, Owner
P.O. Box 4158
Santa Fe, NM 87502
Phone: (800) 497-9516 or (505) 982-2688
Website: http://cutcat.com

Sprite Industries, Inc.
1791 Railroad Street
Corona, CA 92880
Phone: (800) 327-9137 or (951) 735-1015
Fax: (951) 735-1016
Website: www.spritewater.com

Ozone Generators and Air Purifiers

The Cutting Edge
Jules Klapper, Owner
P.O. Box 4158
Santa Fe, NM 87502
Phone: (800) 497-9516 or (505) 982-2688
Website: http://cutcat.com

Reference Material

Gerson Books & Booklets
Material in Support of Gerson Therapy
Available at www.gersonmedia.com

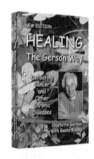

Healing the Gerson Way, Charlotte Gerson and Beata Bishop, 2nd edition (Carmel, CA: Gerson Health Media, 2009). A complete guide to the theory and practice of the Gerson Therapy, developed over 90 years ago by Dr. Max Gerson, MD (1881-1959), *Healing the Gerson Way* is a well-written, easy-to-understand guide that shows how an increasingly toxic, chemically laden, nutritionally empty, modern diet is the main cause of today's worsening health crisis, and offers a brilliant solution in the form of an effective nutritional program that eliminates the underlying causes of disease. This book is also available with *The Beautiful Truth* DVD bound into the back of the book, or with *The Gerson Movie Collection* on Blu-ray, including *The Gerson Miracle, The Beautiful Truth* and *Dying to Have Known* all on one Blu-ray disc.

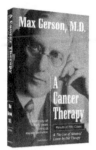

A Cancer Therapy: Results of Fifty Cases and The Cure of Advanced Cancer by Diet Therapy: A Summary of Thirty Years of Clinical Experimentation, 6th ed., Max Gerson, MD (San Diego, CA: Gerson Institute, 2002). Dr. Gerson's seminal work on his cancer therapy, developed over 35 years of clinical experience.

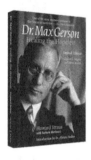

Dr. Max Gerson: Healing the Hopeless, Howard Straus (Carmel, CA: Totality Books, 2009). The official biography of Dr. Max Gerson, chronicling his life and the intertwined development of his therapy, flight from the Nazi Holo-

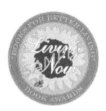

caust, and struggle against American allopathic medicine. In 2013, *Dr. Max Gerson: Healing the Hopeless* won the gold Evergreen Medal for Health and Wellness award from Living Now Book Awards. For more information, please visit www.livingnow-awards.com/about.php.

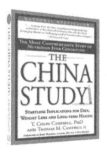

The China Study: Startling Implications for Diet, Weight Loss and Long-term Health, T. Colin Campbell and Thomas M. Campbell II (Dallas: BenBella Books, 2005). One of the world's leading nutritionist sets out his tightly reasoned, experimentally proven case for avoiding animal products, the #1 carcinogen in the world.

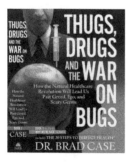

Thugs, Drugs and the War on Bugs: How the Natural Healthcare Revolution Will Lead Us Past Greed, Ego, and Scary Germs, Dr. Brad Case (Prunedale, CA: New Renaissance Books, 2010). A scathing exposé on America's "Sick Care" industry.

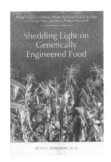

Shedding Light on Genetically Engineered Food: What You Don't Know About the Food You're Eating and What You Can Do to Protect Yourself, Beth Harrison (Lincoln, NE: iUniverse, Inc., 2007). Four-time award-winning book, a stunning eye-opener! This book reveals information you need to know that you won't find in the mainstream media, and delves into how some of the top corporations that control your food have repeatedly done business at the expense of public health. It tells the truth about genetically engineered (GE) food, and how and why you have been kept in the dark about it. The book also outlines what foods to avoid and how you can take action in getting involved with organizations that are advocating for public health.

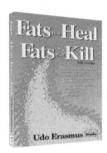

Fats That Heal, Fats That Kill: The Complete Guide to Fats, Oils, Cholesterol and Human Health, Udo Erasmus (Summertown, TN: Alive Books, 1993). Get the skinny on fats! The most current research on common and less well-known oils with therapeutic potential, including flaxseed oil, olive oil, fish oil, evening primrose oil and more. The manufacturing processes that turn healing fats into killing fats explains the effects of these damaging fats on human health, and furnishes information that enables you to choose health-promoting oils.

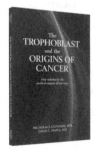

The Trophoblast and the Origins of Cancer: One solution to the medical enigma of our time, Nicholas Gonzales MD (New York: New Spring Press, 2009). This groundbreaking analysis reveals how, more than 100 years ago, the English scientist Dr. John Beard uncovered not only the likely origins of his underlying theory from the perspective of contemporary molecular biology and explores his pioneering use of pancreatic enzymes for cancer treatment. This book also showcases a series of case histories, describing cancer patients successfully treated with pancreatic enzymes by Dr. Gonzalez and Dr. Linda Isaacs (Dr. Gonzalez's partner and coauthor).

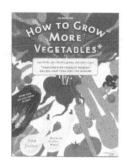

How to Grow More Vegetables Than You Ever Thought Possible on Less Land Than You Can Imagine, John Jeavons (Emeryville, CA: Ten Speed Press, 1995). A classic in the field of sustainable gardening, this book shows how to produce a beautiful, organic garden with minimal watering and care, whether it's just a few tomatoes in a tiny backyard or enough food to feed a family of four on less than half an acre. It explains the "grow biointensive" sustainable mini-farming method of gardening, and describes a complete general approach to gardening, including soil preparation, bed preparation, fertilizations, composting, seed propagation, transplanting, crop rotation, watering and weeding. It contains information for beginning, intermediate and advanced gardeners, including master charts for specific foods and plants to maximize the effectiveness of time and space in the smallest-scale growing area and sample garden plans. Recommends companion plants and methods of natural pest control.

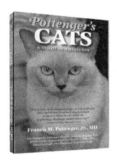

Pottenger's Cats: A Study in Nutrition, Francis Pottenger (Lemon Grove, CA: Price Pottenger Nutrition Foundation, 1995). Dr. Francis M. Pottenger, Jr., was an original thinker and keen observer whose imagination, integrity and common sense gave him the courage to question official dogma. Dedicated to the cause of preventing chronic illness, he made significant contributions to the understanding of the role of nutrition in maintaining good health.

In his classical experiments in cat feeding, more than 900 cats were studied over 10 years. Dr. Pottenger found that only diets containing raw milk and raw meat produced optimal health: good bone structure and density, wide palates with plenty of space for teeth, shiny fur, no parasites or disease, reproductive ease and gentleness.

Cooking the meat or substituting heat-processed milk for raw resulted in heterogeneous reproduction and physical degeneration, increasing with each generation. Vermin and parasites abounded. Skin diseases and allergies increased from 5% to over 90%. Bones became soft and pliable. Cats suffered from adverse personality changes, hypothyroidism and most of the degenerative diseases encountered in human medicine. They died out completely by the fourth generation.

The changes Pottenger observed in cats on the deficient diets paralleled the human degeneration that Dr. Price found in tribes that had abandoned traditional diets.

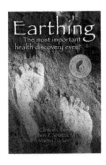

Earthing: The Most Important Health Discovery Ever?, Clint Ober, Stephen Sinatra MD and veteran health writer Martin Zucker (Laguna Beach, CA: Basic Health Publications, 2010). The surface of the Earth resonates with natural, subtle energies. Ongoing scientific research is discovering the details as to why people feel significantly better when they connect with these omnipresent energy fields. "Earthing" refers to the process of connecting by walking barefoot outside—as humans have done throughout history—or sitting, working or sleeping grounded indoors. For more than a decade, thousands of people around the world—men, women, children and athletes—have incorporated Earthing into their daily routines and report that they sleep better, have less pain and stress and recover faster from trauma. Earthing immediately equalizes your body to the same energy level, or potential, as the Earth. This results in synchronizing your internal biological clocks, hormonal cycles and physiological rhythms, and suffusing your body with healing, negatively charged free electrons abundantly present on the surface of the Earth. Earthing is among the most natural and safest things you can do. Sleeping grounded is the best way to reap the benefits of connecting with the Earth.

NEW for 2014
Lose Weight the Gerson Way (available Fall 2015)

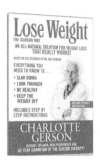

Lose Weight the Gerson Way (Carmel, CA: Gerson Health Media, 2012)

• Slim down

• Look younger

• Live longer

• Be healthy

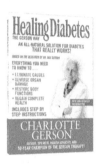

Healing Diabetes the Gerson Way (Carmel, CA: Gerson Health Media, 2012)

• Eliminate causes

• Reverse organ damage

• Restore body functions

• Regain complete health

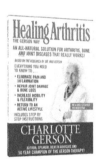

Healing Arthritis the Gerson Way (Carmel, CA: Gerson Health Media, 2012)

• Eliminate pain and inflammation

• Repair joint damage

• Increase mobility and flexibility

• Return to an active lifestyle

HEALING BOOKLETS by Charlotte Gerson (Carmel, CA: Cancer Research Wellness Institute, 2002), 30 pages each. This is a series of nine booklets, eight of which detail the reason why cancer occurs, how and why the Gerson Therapy heals, a short outline of the Gerson Therapy and about a dozen stories of recovered patients. The ninth booklet covers "auto-immune" diseases."

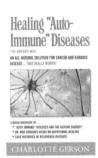

Healing "Auto-Immune" Diseases: The Gerson Way. This booklet introduces Dr. Max Gerson and reviews the foundation of the Gerson Therapy, that cancer and most chronic diseases are able to manifest in the body because of toxicity and nutritional deficiency. Charlotte Gerson gives an overview of the Gerson Therapy and reviews some of the methods used in the program. Also included are factual case histories of individuals confronted with "auto-immune" disease, such as Crohn's disease, ulcerative colitis, multiple sclerosis, rheumatoid arthritis, and chronic fatigue, and how they overcame them using the Gerson Therapy.

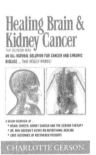

Healing Brain & Kidney Cancer: The Gerson Way. This booklet introduces Dr. Max Gerson and reviews the founding principle of the Gerson Therapy, that cancer and most chronic diseases are able to manifest in the body because of toxicity and nutritional deficiency. Charlotte Gerson gives an overview of the Gerson Therapy and reviews some of the methods used in the program.Also included are factual case histories of individuals confronted with life-threatening diseases, such as brain and kidney cancer, and how they overcame them using the Gerson Therapy.

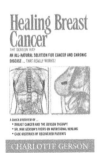

Healing Breast Cancer: The Gerson Way. This booklet introduces Dr. Max Gerson and the foundation of the Gerson Therapy, that cancer and most chronic diseases are able to manifest in the body because of toxicity and nutritional deficiency. Charlotte Gerson gives an overview of the Gerson Therapy and reviews some of the methods used in the program. Also included are factual case histories of individuals confronted with breast cancer and their stories of recovery using the Gerson Therapy.

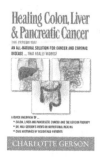

Healing Colon, Liver and Pancreatic Cancer: The Gerson Way. This booklet introduces Dr. Max Gerson and reviews the founding principle of the Gerson Therapy, that cancer and most chronic diseases are able to manifest in the body because of toxicity and nutritional deficiency. Charlotte Gerson gives an overview of the Gerson Therapy and reviews some of the methods used in the program. Also included are case histories of individuals confronted with colon, liver and pancreatic cancer and how they overcame them using the Gerson Therapy.

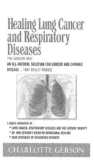

Healing Lung Cancer and Respiratory Diseases: The Gerson Way. This booklet introduces Dr. Max Gerson and the foundation of the Gerson Therapy, that cancer and most chronic diseases are able to manifest in the body because of toxicity and nutritional deficiency. Charlotte Gerson gives an overview of the Gerson Therapy and reviews some of the methods used in the program. Also included are case histories of individuals confronted with lung cancer and other respiratory diseases and how they overcame them using the Gerson Therapy.

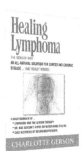

Healing Lymphoma: The Gerson Way. This booklet introduces Dr. Max Gerson and the foundation of the Gerson Therapy, that cancer and most chronic diseases are able to manifest in the body because of toxicity and nutritional deficiency. Charlotte Gerson gives an overview of the Gerson Therapy and reviews some of the methods used in the program. Also included are factual case histories of individuals confronted with lymphoma and how they overcame it using the Gerson Therapy.

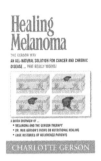

Healing Melanoma: The Gerson Way. This booklet introduces Dr. Max Gerson and the founding principle of the Gerson Therapy, that melanoma and most chronic diseases are able to manifest in the body because of toxicity and nutritional deficiency. Charlotte Gerson gives an overview of the Gerson Therapy and reviews some of the methods used in the program. Also included are case histories of individuals confronted with melanoma and how they overcame them using the Gerson Therapy.

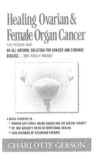

Healing Ovarian & Female Organ Cancer: The Gerson Way. This booklet introduces Dr. Max Gerson and the foundation of the Gerson Therapy, that cancer and most chronic diseases are able to manifest in the body because of toxicity and nutritional deficiency. Charlotte Gerson gives an overview of the Gerson Therapy and reviews some of the methods used in the program. Also included are factual case histories of individuals confronted with ovarian and female organ cancer and how they overcame them using the Gerson Therapy.

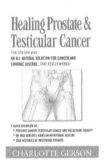

Healing Prostate & Testicular Cancer: The Gerson Way. This booklet introduces Dr. Max Gerson and the foundation of the Gerson Therapy, that cancer and most chronic diseases are able to manifest in the body because of toxicity and nutritional deficiency. Charlotte Gerson gives an overview of the Gerson Therapy and reviews some of the methods used in the program, with a focus on prostate and testicular cancer. Also included are factual case histories of individuals confronted with either prostate or testicular cancer and how they overcame it using the Gerson Therapy.

COMING SOON

- *Healing the Gerson Way*, 3rd edition

Gerson Movies & DVDs
Other Materials in Support of the Gerson Therapy

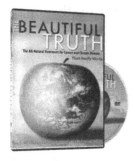

The Beautiful Truth (2008). Cinematographer Stephen Kroschel's third feature-length Gerson documentary. A teen embarks on a cross-country trip to investigate the merits of a natural therapy for cancer based upon diet. He learns that this cure, which boldly contradicts the treatments promoted by the medical establishment, has existed for over half a century.

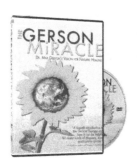

The Gerson Miracle, Stephen Kroschel (2004). Winner of the 2004 Golden Palm for "Best Picture," Beverly Hills Film Festival, Beverly Hills, CA.

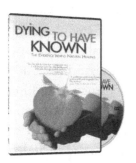

Dying to Have Known, Stephen Kroschel (2006). Awarded Honorable Mention, Feature-length documentary category, 2006 New York International Independent Film and Video Festival, New York City, NY.

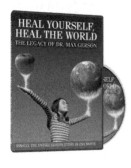

Heal Yourself, Heal the World—The Legacy of Dr. Max Gerson (2013). Finally, all of the Gerson information in one movie! Join Howard Straus (author, scientist, son of Charlotte Gerson and grandson of Dr. Max Gerson) for an in-depth examination of the Gerson Therapy—how it works, the science behind it and why it works. The life story of Dr. Gerson, his development of the life-saving Gerson Therapy and the information regarding why it works, the benefits of using it and a quick overview of how to implement it is just so big that previously it could only be related in a trilogy of films. *Heal Yourself, Heal the World* is a new review of the Gerson Therapy and, for this retelling of the story, we created an attention-grabbing script and intertwined the best parts from the other films with new interviews, updated scientific information, modern graphics and even media from Dr. Gerson's time. *Heal Yourself, Heal the World* includes:

- Historical information on Dr. Max Gerson never before presented on film

- In-depth explanations from scientists, researchers and nutritional experts on the science behind the Gerson Therapy and why it works

- Reports from doctors who use the Gerson Therapy to heal their patients

- Personal stories from Gerson patients who healed themselves of cancer and other diseases using the Gerson Therapy

Special features:

- The original 1946 broadcast by popular radio reporter Raymond Gram Swing, who detailed the congressional testimony of Dr. Max Gerson and the benefits of his then revolutionary new method of treating cancer and disease

- A downloadable and printable PDF of Dr. Gerson's original testimony before the Pepper–Neely congressional subcommittee that was considering a $100 million appropriations bill for the study and treatment of cancer (a rare torical document because Dr. Gerson's testimony was later removed from congressional archives)

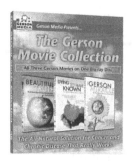

The Gerson Movie Collection (2012). This collection contains **three original Gerson movies ALL ON ONE BLU-RAY DISC:**

- *The Beautiful Truth*
- *Dying to Have Known*
- *The Gerson Miracle*

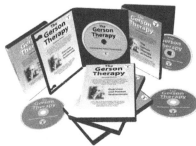

The Gerson Therapy at Home Series (Four Disc Set) (2010). Watching this complete DVD set will provide a more thorough understanding of how the therapy works, methods for home application and everyday practicality of the Gerson Therapy. Each volume contains lectures presented by Charlotte Gerson describing topics ranging from the history of the therapy to enema procedure to juicing techniques. The DVDs complement material presented in *Healing The Gerson Way* and offer a visual representation for ideas overviewed in the book.

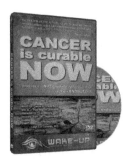

CANCER is Curable NOW (2010). This film might be the breakthrough that brings alternative cancer treatment to the mainstream audience. This documentary brings together more than 30 international, holistic professionals—doctors, scientists, researchers and writers from around the world—who have been working passionately in the field of cancer alternatives. You've probably heard about many of them in books and on TV, but if you'd like to see their knowledge explained in a 90-minute firework display of insights, this movie is the place to do it.

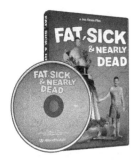

Fat Sick & Nearly Dead (www.jointhereboot.com) (2011). One hundred pounds overweight, loaded up on steroids and suffering from a debilitating autoimmune disease, Joe Cross is at the end of his rope and the end of his hope. In the mirror, he saw a 310-pound man whose gut was bigger than a beach ball and a path laid out before him that wouldn't end well; with one foot already in the grave, the other wasn't far behind. *Fat Sick & Nearly Dead* is an inspiring film that chronicles Joe's personal mission to regain his health.

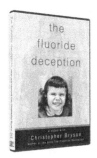

The Fluoride Deception (2012). This short film contains the history of water fluoridation in America. Buy it, free your mind, then ask why the media has fallen silent on this public health crisis. Water fluoridation is killing America. Don't stand for it any longer. In this video, award-winning journalist Christopher Bryson examines "one of the great secret narratives of the industrial era; how fluoride, a grim workplace poison and the most damaging environmental pollutant of the cold war, was added to our drinking water and toothpaste."

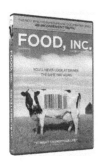

Food, Inc. (2008). For most Americans, the ideal meal is fast, cheap and tasty. *Food, Inc.* examines the costs of putting value and convenience over nutrition and environmental impact.

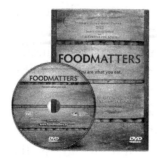

Foodmatters (2008). *"Let thy Food be thy Medicine and thy Medicine be thy Food"*—Hippocrates. That is the message from the founding father of modern medicine, echoed in the controversial new documentary film *Foodmatters* from producer/directors James Colquhoun and Laurentine Ten Bosch. The focus of the film is to help us rethink the belief systems fed to us by our modern medical and health care establishments.

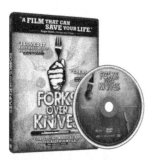

Forks Over Knives (2011). What has happened to us? Despite the most advanced medical technology in the world, we are sicker than ever by nearly every measure. Two out of every three of us are overweight. Cases of diabetes are exploding, especially amongst our younger population. About half of us are taking at least one prescription drug. Major medical operations have become routine, helping to drive health care costs to astronomical levels. Heart disease, cancer and stroke are the country's three leading causes of death, even though billions are spent each year to "battle" these very conditions. Millions suffer from a host of other degenerative diseases. Could it be that there's a single solution to all of these problems—a solution so comprehensive but so utterly straightforward that it's mind-boggling that more of us haven't taken it seriously?

Forks Over Knives examines the profound claim that most, if not all, of the so-called "diseases of affluence" that afflict us can be controlled, or even reversed, by rejecting our present menu of animal-based and processed foods. The major storyline in the film traces the personal journeys of a pair of pioneering yet underappreciated researchers, Dr. T. Colin Campbell, Nutritional Scientist at Cornell University, and Dr. Caldwell Esselstyn, Cardiac Surgeon, Head of Breast Cancer Task Force at Cleveland Clinic.

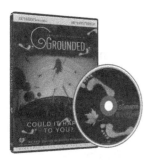

Grounded (2013). This movie tells the true tale of an Alaskan wildlife filmmaker's persistent curiosity and quest to test the claims of what appears to be an outrageously simple and too-good-to-be-true healing concept physical, bare-skin contact with the Earth, which may have been known by civilizations throughout history. New research has started to confirm the unexpected: the surface of the Earth has healing power, like a gigantic treatment table. He introduces this concept to his fellow townsmen in Haines, Alaska (population 1,700), many of who suffer from major pain or disabling conditions. Starting with his own pain relief, he witnesses and films a surprising and miraculous healing in the town generated by simply grounding people to the Earth; that is, reconnecting them to the Earth's healing energy. Even an orphaned moose calf named Karen participates in the healing. The news of the town's response draws the attention of Apollo astronauts who walked on the moon, as well as doctors and scientists. This highly unusual and eye-opening movie premiered on many media platforms, beginning in October 2013. It will change the way you look at the Earth beneath your feet!

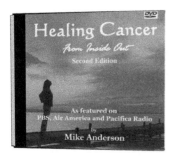

Healing Cancer from The Inside Out (2008). *If you think conventional treatments cure cancer . . . If you think diet cannot cure cancer . . . Think again!*

Part 1, Curing Cancer: The first half of this film deals with the failings of conventional cancer treatments and shows how conventional medicine wildly—and deceptively— exaggerates the benefits of treatments while minimizing the risks. It will provide you with the information you need to accurately assess the risks and benefits of any treatment and speak intelligently to your doctor about such treatments. There is also a section on the "Cancer Industry," which explains the history behind cancer treatments, the suppression of alternative treatments and why chemotherapy, radiation and surgery are the only treatments available to mainstream medicine.

Part 2, Healing Cancer: The second half shows how cancer can be successfully healed with dietary treatments and natural supplementation. It explains common misconceptions about cancer, shows how diets designed to fight cancer are more successful than conventional treatments, discusses startling cancer research findings with T. Colin Campbell (*The China Study*) and has interviews with people who have reversed cancers using diet. It also discusses supplementation and why attitude is important in reversing not only cancer but any disease.

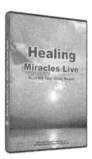

Healing Miracle Live **(3 DVD set)** (2010).

• *5 Steps to Health, Happiness & Sustainability,* Dr. Leonard Horowitz

• *Unleashing Your Inner Healer,* Mike Adams, the Health Ranger

• *Curing the Incurables,* Charlotte Gerson

• *Reversing Diabetes and Heart Disease,* Julian Whitaker, MD. Don't miss (and listen carefully) to Dr. Whitaker's urgent warning to everyone at the end of his presentation.

• *All Juiced Up!* with Jay Kordich, the Father of Juicing

Articles by Dr. Max Gerson
(free PDFs available at www.gersonmedia.com)

1957 "Can Cancer be Prevented?"

1956 "The Cure of Advanced Cancer by Diet Therapy"

1955 "The Gerson Treatment for Cancer"

1949 "Effects of a Combined Dietary Regime on Patients With Malignant Tumors"

1948 "The Jew and Diet"

1946 "Case Histories of Ten Cancer Patients: Clinical Observations Theoretical Considerations and Summary"

1945 "Dietary Considerations in Malignant Neoplastic Diseases"

1943 "Some Aspects of the Problem of Fatigue"

1941 "Feeding the German Army"

1931   "Opening Discussion Modern Dietetic Problems in the Treatment of Tuberculosis, Journal of State Medicine"

Articles by doctors, researchers, specialists and journalists (free PDFs available at www.gersonmedia.com)

2011   "Fluoride Poisoning—It's All Over," Mary Sparrowdancer
2011   "New Study: Fluoride Can Damage the Brain—Avoid Use in Children," *PR Newswire*, New York. June 21, 2011. Quotes study in *Neurologia*.
2010   "The Philosophy of Living Foundation Interviews Howard Straus on the Naturalised Sum Reversal of Cancer," Alexander Rai, October 2010. (Note: Howard is Charlotte Gerson's son and Dr. Max Gerson's grandson)

There are 20 other documents in German and one in Japanese available on the website.

Available through the Gerson Institute (www.gerson.org)

The Cancer Industry: Unraveling the Politics, Ralph W. Moss (New York: Paragon House, 1989). An exposé of the money and power politics, which drives the industry that it treats and victimizes the cancer patient.

Questioning Chemotherapy, Ralph W. Moss (Brooklyn: Equinox Press, 2000). An analysis of the practice and results of chemotherapy, and the reasons behind its widespread use despite its dismal record.

Death by Modern Medicine, Carolyn Dean, MD (Belleville, Ontario: Matrix Vérité, 2005). Dr. Dean painstakingly gathered government statistics and medical journal data, and published information to show that the #1 killer in the United States is ... our medical system.

Living Proof: A Medical Mutiny, Michael Gearin-Tosh (London: Simon & Schuster UK, Ltd., 2002). An Oxford Don, faced with certain death from multiple myeloma or its allopathic treatments, chooses instead to use the Gerson Therapy and Chinese meditation, and survives his prognosis by over 10 years. Witty, incisive and readable.

Fats & Oils, Udo Erasmus (Vancouver, BC: Alive Books, January 1989). The definitive book on fats and oils, and their structures, sources, uses and effects on human health and physiology. Excellent reference.

Fluoride: the Aging Factor, John Yiamouyiannis (Delaware, OH: Health Action Press, 1993). A survey of the suppressed literature on fluoridation of water, vitamins, toothpaste and dental treatments. Chilling and vital information to protect your health and that of your loved ones.

What Really Causes Schizophrenia, Harold D. Foster (Victoria, BC: Trafford Publishing, 2003). Professor Foster presents a novel analysis of the sources and cure of schizophrenia, viewing it as a deficiency or nutritional problem rather than a mental defect.

What Really Causes AIDS, Harold D. Foster (Victoria, BC: Trafford Publishing, 2002). Professor Foster shows the true cause of AIDS as a deficiency of selenium and that it is curable with the proper diet plus selenium supplementation.

Author Index

Subject Index

Item	Qty.	Price	Extended
BOOKS			
Healing the Gerson Way	____	$24.95	____
Healing Arthritis the Gerson Way	____	$17.95	____
Healing Diabetes the Gerson Way	____	$17.95	____
Healing High Blood Pressure the Gerson Way	____	$17.95	____
Dr. Max Gerson: Healing the Hopeless, Second Edition	____	$21.95	____
DVDs and BLU-RAY			
The Beautiful Truth DVD	____	$9.95	____
Dying to Have Known DVD	____	$9.95	____
The Gerson Miracle DVD	____	$9.95	____
Heal Yourself, Heal the World	____	$12.95	____
The Gerson Movie Collection on Blu-ray	____	$9.95	____
BOOKLETS			
Healing Breast Cancer the Gerson Way	____	$4.95	____
Healing Prostate and Testicular Cancer the Gerson Way	____	$4.95	____
Healing Ovarian and Female Organ Cancer the Gerson Way	____	$4.95	____
Healing Colon, Liver and Pancreas Cancer the Gerson Way	____	$4.95	____
Healing Lung Cancer & Respiratory Diseases the Gerson Way	____	$4.95	____
Healing Lymphoma the Gerson Way	____	$4.95	____
Healing Melanoma the Gerson Way	____	$4.95	____
Healing Brain and Kidney Cancer the Gerson Way	____	$4.95	____
Healing "Auto-immune" Diseases the Gerson Way	____	$4.95	____
Subtotal			____
* Shipping/handling			____
9% sales tax (California residents only)			____
Total			____

*   *U.S. only shipping charge of $4 per book, $2 per DVD and $1.25 per booklet. This is an estimated shipping/ handling charge. Actual charge will be calculated by Gerson Health Media. Federal Express charges extra for next-day deliveries for orders placed on Friday.*

To receive a special discount on all items, or sign up for our free email newsletter, please go to http://www.gersonmedia.com.

PERSONAL CHECKS AND MAJOR CREDIT CARDS ACCEPTED.

Name _____

Street Address _____

City/State/Zip _____

Phone_____E-mail_____

Credit Card Number _____ Exp. Date_____

Gerson Health Media
859 Washington Street, #202, Red Bluff, CA 96080
(530) 529-1100 • bill@gersonmedia.com • www.gersonmedia.com

Available from Gerson Health Media (use order form on overleaf)

 Healing the Gerson Way, Charlotte Gerson with Beata Bishop. Based on the research of Dr. Max Gerson, this well-written, easy-to-understand, how-to guide for using the Gerson Therapy shows you how to overcome cancer and chronic disease. Also included are hints and tips, and more than 90 pages of Gerson-approved recipes.

.... **$24.95**

 Healing Arthritis the Gerson Way, Charlotte Gerson. A complete how-to guide for repairing and reversing arthritic conditions using the well-known Gerson Therapy. Written in an easy-to-read style, it includes the latest medical research on arthritis and updated information on the most common forms of the disease.

.... **$17.95**

 Healing Diabetes the Gerson Way, Charlotte Gerson. This book provides a powerful program to reverse type 2 diabetes and return you to complete health. It offers an easy-to-follow, how-to guide for using the Gerson Therapy to overcome type 2 diabetes, and the simple, step-by-step instructions guide you through the program.

.... **$17.95**

 Healing High Blood Pressure the Gerson Way, Charlotte Gerson. A complete how-to guide for rapidly reversing high blood pressure (hypertension) using the well-known Gerson Therapy. Learn why you have high blood pressure, what its devastating results can be and how to ban it from your life forever.

.... **$17.95**

 Dr. Max Gerson: Healing the Hopeless, by Howard Straus with Barbara Marinacci. Inspiring and uplifting biography of the originator of the Gerson Therapy, chronicling Dr. Gerson's life, development of his world-famous dietary therapy, flight from the Nazi Holocaust and successful search for a holistic and effective treatment for cancer.

.... **$21.95**

 The Beautiful Truth DVD, Stephen Kroschel. Follow Garrett on a cross-country road trip to investigate the Gerson Therapy. He meets with cancer survivors who present their stories of triumph and healing by following the Gerson Therapy, and interviews scientists, doctors and researchers who discuss the multibillion dollar medical industry.

.... **$9.95**

 Dying to Have Known DVD, Stephen Kroschel. Hear the testimonies of patients, scientists, surgeons and nutritionists who testify to the Gerson Therapy's efficacy in reversing cancer and other degenerative diseases and present hard, scientific proof to back up their claims. Testimonies include a Japanese medical school professor who cured himself of liver cancer over 20 years ago.

.... **$9.95**

 The Gerson Miracle DVD, Stephen Kroschel. This film introduces Dr. Max Gerson, who developed a proven remedy for cancer and most chronic and degenerative diseases more than 80 years ago. The Gerson Therapy employs a diet and detoxification regimen to rebuild the immune system and restore the body's own ability to heal itself.

.... **$9.95**

 Heal Yourself Heal the World is a new review of the Gerson Therapy and, for this retelling of the story, we created an attention-grabbing script and intertwined the best parts of other films with new interviews, updated scientific information, modern graphics and even media from Dr. Gerson's time.

.... **$12.95**

 The Gerson Movie Collection on Blu-ray. All three Gerson movies on one Blu-ray disc:
• The Beautiful Truth
• Dying to Have Known
• The Gerson Miracle

.... **$9.95**

 Gerson Health Media
859 Washington Street, #202, Red Bluff, CA 96080
(530) 529-1100 • bill@gersonmedia.com • www.gersonmedia.com

Item	Qty.	Price	Extended
BOOKS			
Healing the Gerson Way	____	$24.95	____
Healing Arthritis the Gerson Way	____	$17.95	____
Healing Diabetes the Gerson Way	____	$17.95	____
Healing High Blood Pressure the Gerson Way	____	$17.95	____
Dr. Max Gerson: Healing the Hopeless, Second Edition	____	$21.95	____
DVDs and BLU-RAY			
The Beautiful Truth DVD	____	$9.95	____
Dying to Have Known DVD	____	$9.95	____
The Gerson Miracle DVD	____	$9.95	____
Heal Yourself, Heal the World	____	$12.95	____
The Gerson Movie Collection on Blu-ray	____	$9.95	____
BOOKLETS			
Healing Breast Cancer the Gerson Way	____	$4.95	____
Healing Prostate and Testicular Cancer the Gerson Way	____	$4.95	____
Healing Ovarian and Female Organ Cancer the Gerson Way	____	$4.95	____
Healing Colon, Liver and Pancreas Cancer the Gerson Way	____	$4.95	____
Healing Lung Cancer & Respiratory Diseases the Gerson Way	____	$4.95	____
Healing Lymphoma the Gerson Way	____	$4.95	____
Healing Melanoma the Gerson Way	____	$4.95	____
Healing Brain and Kidney Cancer the Gerson Way	____	$4.95	____
Healing "Auto-immune" Diseases the Gerson Way	____	$4.95	____
Subtotal			____
***** Shipping/handling			____
9% sales tax (California residents only)			____
Total			____

* *U.S. only shipping charge of $4 per book, $2 per DVD and $1.25 per booklet. This is an estimated shipping/ handling charge. Actual charge will be calculated by Gerson Health Media. Federal Express charges extra for next-day deliveries for orders placed on Friday.*

To receive a special discount on all items, or sign up for our free email newsletter, please go to http://www.gersonmedia.com.

PERSONAL CHECKS AND MAJOR CREDIT CARDS ACCEPTED.

Name _____

Street Address _____

City/State/Zip _____

Phone_____E-mail_____

Credit Card Number _____ Exp. Date_____

Gerson Health Media
859 Washington Street, #202, Red Bluff, CA 96080
(530) 529-1100 • bill@gersonmedia.com • www.gersonmedia.com

Available from Gerson Health Media

(use order form on overleaf)

Healing the Gerson Way, Charlotte Gerson with Beata Bishop. Based on the research of Dr. Max Gerson, this well-written, easy-to-understand, how-to guide for using the Gerson Therapy shows you how to overcome cancer and chronic disease. Also included are hints and tips, and more than 90 pages of Gerson-approved recipes.
.... **$24.95**

Healing Arthritis the Gerson Way, Charlotte Gerson. A complete how-to guide for repairing and reversing arthritic conditions using the well-known Gerson Therapy. Written in an easy-to-read style, it includes the latest medical research on arthritis and updated information on the most common forms of the disease.
.... **$17.95**

Healing Diabetes the Gerson Way, Charlotte Gerson. This book provides a powerful program to reverse type 2 diabetes and return you to complete health. It offers an easy-to-follow, how-to guide for using the Gerson Therapy to overcome type 2 diabetes, and the simple, step-by-step instructions guide you through the program.
.... **$17.95**

Healing High Blood Pressure the Gerson Way, Charlotte Gerson. A complete how-to guide for rapidly reversing high blood pressure (hypertension) using the well-known Gerson Therapy. Learn why you have high blood pressure, what its devastating results can be and how to ban it from your life forever.
.... **$17.95**

Dr. Max Gerson: Healing the Hopeless, by Howard Straus with Barbara Marinacci. Inspiring and uplifting biography of the originator of the Gerson Therapy, chronicling Dr. Gerson's life, development of his world-famous dietary therapy, flight from the Nazi Holocaust and successful search for a holistic and effective treatment for cancer.
.... **$21.95**

The Beautiful Truth DVD, Stephen Kroschel. Follow Garrett on a cross-country road trip to investigate the Gerson Therapy. He meets with cancer survivors who present their stories of triumph and healing by following the Gerson Therapy, and interviews scientists, doctors and researchers who discuss the multibillion dollar medical industry.
.... **$9.95**

Dying to Have Known DVD, Stephen Kroschel. Hear the testimonies of patients, scientists, surgeons and nutritionists who testify to the Gerson Therapy's efficacy in reversing cancer and other degenerative diseases and present hard, scientific proof to back up their claims. Testimonies include a Japanese medical school professor who cured himself of liver cancer over 20 years ago.
.... **$9.95**

The Gerson Miracle DVD, Stephen Kroschel. This film introduces Dr. Max Gerson, who developed a proven remedy for cancer and most chronic and degenerative diseases more than 80 years ago. The Gerson Therapy employs a diet and detoxification regimen to rebuild the immune system and restore the body's own ability to heal itself.
.... **$9.95**

Heal Yourself Heal the World is a new review of the Gerson Therapy and, for this retelling of the story, we created an attention-grabbing script and intertwined the best parts of other films with new interviews, updated scientific information, modern graphics and even media from Dr. Gerson's time.
.... **$12.95**

The Gerson Movie Collection on Blu-ray. All three Gerson movies on one Blu-ray disc:
• The Beautiful Truth
• Dying to Have Known
• The Gerson Miracle
.... **$9.95**

Gerson Health Media
859 Washington Street, #202, Red Bluff, CA 96080
(530) 529-1100 • bill@gersonmedia.com • www.gersonmedia.com